Dedication

For Ted

Contents

Preface

Ironically, although a woman who has had breast cancer
today has a better than 80 percent chance of recovery if
she gets appropriate treatment, we rarely hear victory
reports. It's the deaths we hear about, as if we breast
cancer survivors are bound to protect our privacy even if that
means we deny some other woman facing the disease the information she needs to face her dilemma squarely.

After my surgery, husbands and sons of the dead came
forward to offer me their support. "I know how difficult this
is for you. My first wife died after a heroic battle." Only one
woman who knew about breast cancer from personal experience told me about it. I needed more friends like her.
Statistics show they're out there, reconstructed or wearing a
prosthesis, glad that nobody knows.

I determined from the beginning to keep a faithful record
and share it. Of course, it was tedious and long. I've tried to
make this stripped-down version user-friendly. I'm not sure I
have succeeded. I wanted to maintain the sense of how I experienced cancer, giving the reader no information I did not
have at the time I wrote each entry. I wanted to keep the im-
mediacy of the present tense, in which I wrote many of my
reactions. This has created a few awkward shifts when one
day's commentary is in present while the next is written in
past tense. I'm pretty sure, though, most readers will be able
to follow these shifts.

In trimming down the journal, I have tried to arrange ma-
terial topically rather than chronologically in order to eliminate repetition. This means that the story does not always
move steadily forward. In places chapters overlap.

Chapter 1

CASHING IN

Actually it's 5:49 a.m. and I've had a good night's sleep—am all slept out. For the past 48 minutes I've been lying in bed, thinking about what I need to do today. This is the day I had planned to do most of a year's accumulated mending before going to my office, but it looks like I'm ready to get back to my cancer journal.

Last evening, pushing my cart around a corner in the Village Market, I met my friend Jeannie Robertson.

"You're back!" I exclaimed. "Tell me about your trip to Russia."

"It was a wonderful trip," Jeannie began, giving me the highlights. And then she asked, "Do you have a new book out?"

"I finished one Friday, and I'm trying to make my line printer work today," I said. "But not the book I was supposed to do this summer." Jeannie knew about the cancer journal.

"I kept a journal in Russia," she gloated. "I never keep journals, but I made myself do it because I knew I'd need it later for information. Of course, writing's not like that for you, but for me it's a real chore."

If Jeannie only knew! I try to explain to students in my classes that writing is always a chore, and the longer we write and the better we write, the harder it is. Just like my

18-year-old freshman composition students, I love to read a piece of my finished work, but I struggle and sweat over paragraphs as they take shape. And without a doubt, this cancer journal has been the most disagreeable chore of all.

When I write stories about other people, I can imagine their disappointments and their griefs. When I finish a chapter, I turn off my mental video and am myself again, quite comfortably distinct and distant from the crisis I've been writing about. In this project, however, I've had to think deeply inside-out instead of outside-in. It's like I told Jeannie last evening, I'm ready now to forget about cancer. When I get dressed in the morning I stuff my tear-shaped Dacron-filled pillow into the left side of my bra, but then for the rest of the day I'm too absorbed in everything else to think about cancer. I don't really want to think about it when I'm feeling so good. It's something I'd just as soon forget.

But if I've learned one thing from having cancer, it is that once you've had it, nothing is the same again. The insurance agent who begged for "just a moment of your valuable time" to explain why you need to buy her health insurance plan suddenly becomes embarrassed and says you are really too high a risk for her company to accept. Little kids who have heard whispers at home stare and wonder which one is a fake. And family members are incredibly thoughtful nearly all the time. Of all the changes cancer brings about, the most significant, it seems to me, is the change in family relationships.

I realize that some husbands bolt and run from a wife who comes home after surgery with a 14-inch scar where her breast used to be. But I rather believe that most men faced with this kind of shock respond as tenderly as my husband has, and breast cancer, instead of blighting a marriage, usually strengthens it. For the very real possibility of death is like a dash of cold water. It wakes up both husband and wife to the fact that whatever living they plan to do, they had better do it now. Whatever love they feel, they had better express it lavishly now.

Now is the word.

This morning my begonias billow over the railing on the kitchen deck, pink and white and deep, deep green. This morning the ripe cantaloupe I've cut for breakfast floods my corner of the kitchen with fragrance so rich I can taste it in the air. And today, when he comes to kiss me before he shaves, Ted's kisses are the sweetest in 28 years of marriage.

I don't plan to die in the near future. I'm not sick. Certainly I'm not. But just knowing that "the enemy" might be alive somewhere in the secret places of my bones or brain makes me value what I have *now* as I wouldn't otherwise.

The year I was in second grade the JMV reading course included a book called *Wild Animals of Africa*. My mother read a chapter aloud every evening—just before sending me upstairs to bed. Every night I got my back up against the wall before Mom turned the light out. As she went downstairs I listened for the animals to creep out of the closet, in from the hall, down from the attic. In the darkness I identified all the predators—hyenas, lions, leopards. I trembled as their breath fluttered the curtains at my window in the moonlight, and I saw their eyes gleaming in the shadows.

I think all fear is like that—irrational. Not that there is nothing to be reasonably afraid of, but that once we start being afraid, even for good reasons, we turn our imaginations loose. Maybe you don't, but I do.

I was waiting for a Monday faculty meeting to begin when Barbara James, a member of the nursing department, came in and sat down beside me. Making conversation and following the foolproof icebreaker of asking advice, I mentioned a health concern to her.

"What should I do?" I ask.

"Get a mammogram," she retorted. "Tomorrow morning at the latest. Erlanger Hospital is Southern College's preferred provider. Go there."

Before noon the following day I was pretty sure I had cancer. All I needed for final confirmation was a biopsy, and the doctor scheduled that within a few days. I went home shaken—about the strangest things. About the garden seeds I wouldn't plant next spring—shaken but relieved at the same time that I hadn't paid $125 for the load of rich soil I had almost ordered for my raised beds. At least if I died before April that money wouldn't be wasted.

"That's providential," I muttered as I got out of the car and reached for my briefcase.

The maple in front of the house looked tattered after a hot, dry September. The red geraniums in the window boxes drooped. I set my briefcase on the porch, turned on the hose, and watered them. The tree's roots were deep in the hillside's soil. It could manage weeks between rains. I turned off the water, coiled the hose, and unlocked the front door.

Inside, I glanced at the new sofa—not fully paid for yet, but covered by an insurance policy that guaranteed it would be paid off if I died.

"That's providential," I said again, thinking of my sister-in-law Nytta, whose husband had dropped life insurance on their mortgage just weeks before he died in an accident.

Then I sat down on the insured sofa and laughed at myself. As if I had God all cased out! As if He were taking better care of me than He took of Nytta! Often enough I had bristled when others explained God's plans for their lives as if they were giving a geometry proof:

"He allowed experience X to happen to me so that I couldn't be discouraged when experience Y happened. And then He gave me trial Z so that . . ."

That kind of reasoning had always seemed like a mixture of speculation and presumption to me, as if any of us can reconstruct God's logic.

I ran my hands over the deep blue velvet of the sofa and tried to stop the internal fidgeting—to be still all the way to the center of my body. One moment I felt scared, and the next I didn't, just rather startled at coming to the edge of things—like coming suddenly to the rim of a canyon and looking down the abyss and across it. I thought about Kate in one of my stories and how as I wrote her story I projected myself into her experience with breast cancer 70 years ago. She'd had no money or medical options. Maybe I had been prompted by Providence to write that story too.

Kate's encounter was part of a book-length narrative I wrote as a thesis for my master's degree. I sat there on the blue sofa thinking about Kate. Then I remembered a conversation with my project director at the university.

"I don't like reading even the best quality short stories," I told my friend and mentor, novelist Ken Smith. "They're too depressing."

14

He had accepted my manuscript and had grudgingly conceded that the true story I had written did indeed fulfill the requirements of good fiction. My characters were complex, the way people are in real life, entangled in conflicts like real life, as a result of the very actions that promised resolution.

"So you think the stories I've assigned you to read are depressing?" Ken said, his deeply furrowed face enigmatic behind his beard. "What about your own stories? Nearly all your work is filled with dark people doing pretty dark things. What's so cheerful about the stories you write?"

"If you're talking about sin and sinners, I agree," I said.

Ken's whiskers puckered around the place where his mouth must be. His eyes looked tired. "Call it whatever you want. It's the disease that makes us all human, and our humanity is all we have to write about."

"You're wrong there," I told him. "We have a Saviour."

Ken shrugged. "And you think that solves everything?" He asked it first and then repeated the words as a statement. "You think that solves everything. If there's a weakness in your writing, Helen, that's it. You insist on resolutions, solutions, happy endings."

He scowled as he concentrated on jotting something in his notebook. When he looked up, his eyes were dismal, and the nervous twitch in his left temple jerked repeatedly. "What makes you so sure of happy endings?" he demanded. "How many happy endings have you lived through?"

"A bunch. More than you'd dream," I said. "And I have good reason to expect more."

Ken shook hands across the table. He closed his notebook. "What puzzles me is that I want to rule out the act of God that provides the easy-out in your stories. But the way you show God at work, it's not an artificial fix up—

more like the natural course things take—as if God were a 'given' in the whole situation."

I was about to reply when Ken added, "Of course, for you, God is 'given.'"

That September afternoon when I learned I had cancer, as I thought of my years writing about other people's troubles, I kicked off my shoes and stretched out on the sofa. The late afternoon sun slanted across the fern in front of the window. The leaves cast lacy shadows on the opposite wall.

The next morning I got up about 4:00, a little earlier than usual, but not much. I pulled on a sweat suit over my nightgown and arranged the throw pillows around me in my usual spot at the end of the sofa. I reached for my Bible and held it in my lap while I began composing myself to pray, expecting some feeling to signal the dramatic, the unusual. Instead, I felt only my Bible, the familiar grain of its cover, its weight in my hands.

I ought to look for some comforting passage, I thought. But I didn't feel at all in need of comforting.

I ought to look for something to give me strength for what lies ahead, I thought, vaguely remembering a quotation I had memorized long ago. Then I laughed. "This is ridiculous, Lord," I admitted. "Now is the future I've been preparing a lifetime for. This is the time to relax and enjoy the benefits of all the time we've spent together through the years. It feels so good to have You here now and to know there's nothing to worry about."

I sat motionless for an hour, satisfied, enjoying the rest before everything started happening. It wasn't that I was certain the surgery would get rid of the cancer or that I would recover after further treatment. But I was certain that I could trust God to manage even the worst case scenario for me.

That day I collected rough drafts of essays from my four college composition classes. Critiquing those papers occupied my attention until I left for the hospital. I hardly thought about having cancer. I certainly didn't feel sick. It was hard to believe I was.

Chapter 2

How We Came to This

I grew up in Minnesota. Which accounts for a lot of things. While just being born there and living there for 24 years doesn't guarantee a rigid spine and a stiff upper lip, it helps. Of course, my ancestors had been toughening up in the climate for several generations, so I inherited a strong constitution. I grew up expecting hardships and physical discomforts. I grew up expecting to survive.

I also grew up loving Jesus and trusting Him. A few years ago in a prayer meeting a friend commented that even for a person who has always been in the church, there has to be a time, a specific moment, when the Christian consciously gives her life to God.

"Yes," I said. "True. Every day." But there never was a time for me when I hadn't begun the day with the same covenant. Not that I was more pious than other children, more obedient or less quarrelsome—just that I loved Jesus, loved Him because He loved me and I knew it. Always had.

I grew up loving books, probably in response to the law of supply and demand—books being scarce and expensive, therefore desirable. I loved words and used them for playthings, composing poems and dialogues while I brought in the cows or picked blueberries, refined the cadences pumping my battered green Schwinn bicycle down the corduroy driveway to the mailbox. Setting my words to music and singing fortissimo. I loved the old literature books Daddy salvaged when a country school disbanded — every few months I started reading with Beowulf and ended with Matthew Arnold, "a young and promising" poet at the time the book was published when my grandfather was in grade school. And Whittier and Lowell, Longfellow and Emerson. I loved the King James Bible. Its rhythms, its pace, its cryptic ambiguities. When I was 11 I read it through for the first time. I've tried to break the Bible year habit in recent years, determined to do something more creative, but I keep it up because it's like eating potatoes and beans and bread. Whatever else there might be to eat, the Bible is "real" food, and I want the whole thing.

So I'm a product of all these, and like anyone else, of a thousand unidentifiable influences.

Ted grew up in Washington State, where his mother taught English at Columbia Academy and served as librarian. We met at Walla Walla College in 1961, both of us members of the English Club and into writing poetry.

I made up my mind to marry Ted the afternoon he asked me to critique his portfolio of poems. Even though I lacked romantic experience, I sensed from his poems that I was destined to be "bone of his bone, flesh of his flesh" but also that he was wary. Nearly six years later we were married. But he was still wary — didn't fully trust me, especially since he wasn't quite sure how he had become a married man. A few months after the wedding we moved to Collegedale, Tennessee, then the following year to Sand Mountain in the corner of Alabama a few miles from

Chattanooga, Tennessee, the big attraction being a thriving church and church school in the country. We started our family immediately—Greg born in 1969, Doug in 1971, and Emily in 1973.

Greg put together his first sentence when he was 11 months old: "I do!" Ten minutes later he yelled, "I did it!" I think I was that kind of infant. My mother says I was. Pushy, independent. It's hard for people like me to be sick.

Ted was teaching fourth grade in those days, but he was about as dedicated to graduate school as to his teaching. He finished an M.Ed. before Doug was born, an M.S. in clinical psychology when Emily was a baby, but never did finish the Ph.D. in educational psychology he started that same fall. I joked that he quit before writing the dissertation because I refused to type it for him. Actually, his health was in trouble because of the years of concentrated study—not enough rest, not enough exercise, too much stress. We both knew that a return to teaching was out of the question. And so we opened a day-care center for the aged sponsored by Jackson County Alabama Pensions and Security Department.

Our clients were mostly women in their 80s, frail but hardly feeble, neighborly by nature but isolated in homes spread across both shoulders of the mountain, lonely. Ted and I had lived there for 10 years, but it was the day-care center that turned us into something that might pass for Southerners.

20

During our 10 years on Sand Mountain we had gone to potlucks and learned to eat crowder peas and purple-hulled peas and silver-hulled peas and corn bread and okra—had learned to eat Southern food and even to cook the way Southerners cook. We had gone to church and taught classes and learned to sing Southern gospel. Our three children talked like natives of Sand Mountain whenever they spoke in public, and people in the Floral Crest Church treated us like neighbors, but we still thought of ourselves as foreigners until we started that center—with no resources and no experience, just the normal human instincts and the love of Jesus.

But our clients were the ones who taught us about loving. These men and women had spent a lifetime planting the same garden plot their grandparents had planted, and then watched their own children become parents and grandparents, still planting the same gardens with okra and beans and purple-hulled peas. No doubt about it. We became wiser from this experience, and we became a part of the community—neighbors in a real sense.

Ted's hearing had been bad for a long time, and he wasn't likely to understand a conversation unless he faced the person talking to him. When he talked to Helen Grant on the phone or even face-to-face, they ended up gesturing wildly and still confusing each other.

One noon while we were gathered around the table for lunch, Granny Rainey, her eyes marbled with cataracts, listened as they tried to untangle the day's misunderstanding. Granny Rainey smiled, showing one bottom incisor, the only tooth she had left.

"Mr. Pyke," she said. "Granny Grant. You'uns ought to see Dr. Ownby. He's great at doctorin' ears. He fixed mine 30 year ago. I hain't had airy a trouble hearin' since."

Ted pushed his chair back from the table. "What did he do for you, Granny?"

"Cleaned out my ears," said Mrs. Rainey in her whispery lisp. "That's what he done."

"What you say?" queried Mrs. Grant loudly.

"Get Dr. Ownby to clean out those ears of yourn, I say," breathed Mrs. Rainey.

Ted looked at me and then at Mrs. Rainey. "Tell us about it."

Granny Rainey clasped her hands on her lap—a lap that had cradled 15 of her own children and countless grandchildren. Mrs. Grant clasped her hands over breasts that had nursed 10 children, the last when she was 54 years old.

"Couldn't hear worth a flip," Granny Rainey began, "so I had Billy take me over to Dr. Ownby's. He just looked in my ears, and he said what they wanted was a good washin' out. Told Mrs. O'Dell. Told her, 'Git a dishpan.' Mrs. O'Dell come with the dishpan, and Dr. Ownby just pulled my head over like so and poured into my ear a whole pitcher of warm water with some kind of soap he mixed up. Just poured the whole business in, and it come out the other ear. 'Turn your head over,' he says then, and he poured another pitcher in that ear to be sure he got it all."

"Oh?" Ted said.

"The earwax."

Around the table withered faces reflected either knowing indulgence or full acceptance of Granny Rainey's account. Dr. Ownby was sacred community property. Sometimes they spent whole afternoons, like fishermen, topping each other's tales of Dr. Ownby's medical miracles.

I foolishly tried to set Mrs. Rainey straight. "But, Granny, that couldn't be. Your ears aren't connected that way. There's no passage between your ears."

"Mine is."

I went for a 1956 fifth grade health book I sometimes used when showing them pictures of their ailing inner parts. I found a four-color diagram of the inner and middle ear with the cochlea and auditory nerve and the brain. "See," I said. "Your brain is between your ears. The water couldn't run all the way through."

Granny Rainey's nearly sightless eyes smiled serenely. "It did."

"But your brain is there," I repeated.

"Mine ain't," she said.

And that was final.

We talked about hernias, bunions, and ingrown toenails. My clients would rather discuss their bowel disorders even than childbirth, and they spent a lot of time with that old health book, speculating on the tangles a person could develop with all those yards of intestines coiled up inside. They looked at the pictures and pointed out the locations of cancers afflicting their kinfolk and neighbors, living and dead.

The 1956 book showed a sexless human anatomy and did not include a picture of the breast. Maybe that's why I don't recall any discussions of breast cancer. Or maybe it was just these women's natural modesty that allowed them to discuss the length of their labors and the number of their confinements, even the current conditions of their wombs when no men were present, but prohibited mentioning external bodily parts above the elbow or ankle. If they had lost mothers or sisters or daughters to breast cancer, they weren't telling.

I had always heard that if a woman nursed all her babies she wouldn't get breast cancer; that breast cancer was somehow related to thwarting Nature's intentions. Even though I had breast-fed Greg and Doug and Emily, I usually checked myself once a month for lumps. I didn't expect ever to find one.

Chapter 3

What Is God Good For?

I feel a little strange living here in Collegedale and attending this church with 2,300 members. I miss Floral Crest Church, where on an ordinary Sabbath about 150 attend. We could hardly bring ourselves to leave our Sabbath school class. But after driving 45 miles to and from work for several years, we realized that we were spending too much time on the freeway. We moved August 1991. Although we are beginning to build friendships with the church and faculty family, I still feel torn from the comfort of familiar windows and faces.

I wake up these autumn mornings expecting to see the pin oak red against the sky, to look out my kitchen windows on the two rows of cedars Ted spared when we cleared the yard 20 years ago, to look out my living room windows where on the east the last frost-touched begonias bank against the vinca minor tumbling over the stone curbing, and on the west beyond the three apricot trees the woods drop away to the ponds. Here in Collegedale I step out onto the deck in the foggy darkness of a rainy night for another look at tulip poplars towering behind the house and up the ridge. I lie in bed an extra half hour some mornings to watch gray squirrels set the boughs dancing against the dawn sky.

Just as we never quite moved from the first home we remember from childhood, so I cannot quite get out of the house where our children were babies, where I struggled with a washing machine that frequently overflowed, where we dug holes and planted things. Today I keep remembering bullfrog tadpoles in the big mud puddle in the tractor road, the airplane with eight-foot wingspan (which Greg built of scrap lumber and insisted he would someday fly), and the thousand-pound raft he wanted me to help him carry through the woods to the pool below the waterfall.

All my life I've spread my roots in deep soil. To most of my students Collegedale seems like the shallowest of backwaters—really out of the mainstream—"Country-country." I guess if they've come here from New York or Atlanta, it is. But for me the current runs pretty fast here. I feel in danger of being uprooted and washed away. This is no place to face a crisis. I ought to be on familiar ground, among my friends.

What I mean is, I feel vulnerable and out of control—not in charge of my own situation. I resist doctors taking charge of me. Not the surgery. I chose the surgery without hesitation. I resist being a child. I feel powerless, stripped of authority. I didn't agree to have cancer. I can't stop it.

Once, before Greg and Doug started school, I had purchased fabric and a pattern for a new dress, but when I got everything out to make it, I discovered there were only a few bent pins in my pincushion.

"Buy me some straight pins on your way home tomorrow," I told Ted.

Maybe because he knew exactly where to find them on the shelf in the school supply store, but more probably because that's just the way he thinks things ought to be done, Ted stopped by P&S and bought a pound of straight pins. The following afternoon my dress was finished, all but the hem, and I settled myself in a chair in the living room with its yards of skirt across my lap and the box of pins on the arm of my chair. The boys were upstairs playing in their room, but eventually they moved into the hallway, buzzed there for several minutes as they gathered their gear for the descent, then came down slowly, like a Slinky toy, one step at a time. I wondered momentarily how many trips it would take them to get all that stuff back up to their room before supper.

A few thumps and a bang. Whatever they had had, they left it all at the foot of the stairs and came empty-handed into the living room. Greg got two books from the shelf behind me, handed one to Doug, and opened the other across the patched knees of his jeans. That lasted maybe 10 minutes while I thought idyllic thoughts about my boys—so beautiful there with the sun warm on the backs of their necks, the trimmed ends of their hair sheening like deep velvet. Then they erupted simultaneously in opposite directions, both ending up at the foot of the stairs among their toys.

I was nearly a third of the way around the skirt, pins in a row between my lips, and pins spaced an inch and a half apart in the fabric, holding the hem, when Doug flew into the room. Now he was an airplane, with his arms spread wide and engine sounds roaring from his chest. I grabbed, but the pin box flew ahead of him as he struck the arm of my chair. Pins showered the carpet. A pound of straight pins, hardly two touching each other, their heads bright silver against the apple green!

"Well," I said.

Doug looked dismayed for a moment, then grinned.

"You'll have to pick them all up," I said as he dashed to Greg in the hallway.

"He will," Greg assured me as the two of them dumped a boxful of their stuff on the doormat.

Doug came back with a large magnet my aunt had given him.

"I tied a string on it," Greg told me. "So it will work faster."

Always methodical, Doug began near the piano at the outer limits of the spray, swinging his magnet slowly while it gathered a comet's tail of pins sweeping up from the floor. Greg was at his elbow with a mixing bowl to strip the pins off before the next sweep. In five minutes the pins were back in the box, which I put on the top of the piano this time.

"How did you think of the magnet?" I asked Doug. I would have been down on my knees for an hour. I would never have thought of the magnet.

"That's what magnets are for," he said. "That's what they do."

I've thought about that experience hundreds of times in the nearly 20 years since—times when I felt dashed by spills and broken glassware; times when I felt like exploding in frustration, not knowing how to pick up the pieces of broken treasures and broken relationships; times when I faced crisis after crisis not knowing where to get hold of the problem—where to begin. And hundreds of times I have found simple solutions, because I remembered how Doug collected the pins simply by letting the magnet do its work. I have thought about where the power is and what it's for.

Now somewhere between 3:00 and 4:00 a.m. I replay the memory in slow motion. I see the magnet swing through the chaos of my feelings, and I see Jesus standing there— like on the fourth day of Creation—one foot on the land and the other on the sea. He doesn't have to prove He's God by performing a miracle for me. He's already established the fact. He's in control, and He has infinite power— and a lot of information I don't have.

Chapter 4

BEFORE THE INCISION

Since I had no classes scheduled for Tuesday, I had no excuse to put off going for the mammogram. Barbara James had told me the previous afternoon that I could just walk into Erlanger's Breast Center, because Erlanger was the college's preferred provider. It was a little more complicated than that, but not much. Ten minutes after I arrived, I was wearing a gown and, along with several other women in the waiting area, was watching a video produced by the American Cancer Society. It provided lots of information about self-examination and how to know what was a lump and what was just natural lumpiness characteristic of some women's breast tissue. But I wasn't checking for a lump. I knew I had one. I picked up several booklets from the table.

Questions and Answers About Breast Lumps. I turned a couple of pages. "Q: What should I do if I find a lump in my breast?" SEE YOUR DOCTOR IMMEDIATELY. I don't have a doctor here. We've just moved. Then followed a list of procedures by which the doctor would evaluate the lump. Palpation. Aspiration. Mammogram. (I was doing this backward.) Biopsy. The booklet said that was the only way to know for certain whether a lump was benign or malignant.

While I knew those words, I could see that I needed the glossary. By the time a technician called me for my mammogram, I had the information in my first booklet under control. Vocabularywise. I found out during the next few minutes that knowing the facts in the abstract is quite different from suspecting the facts have become personal.

First, routine mammograms of both sides. Back to the waiting area while a radiologist examined the film.

"Routine," the technician assured me, "in all cases where a woman has discovered a lump herself."

Twenty minutes later, numerous more mammograms of the left side. Back to the waiting area. Wait for the radiologist again. More mammograms. More readings. Finally instructions that I need to see my doctor, who will tell me just what has been found.

Not panic, but definite palpitations in my heart. I gave them the name of the college physician. When I reached his office, he had not yet received the information. He got on the phone and asked for it. He examined me and scolded me about not coming sooner.

Several weeks before, I had noticed some soreness and swelling in my left breast, not a lump, but a tender place as if I had bruised myself. I wasn't concerned, because I had been packing heavy boxes, lifting them, carrying them, shoving furniture around—getting ready to move. Yes, I had just bruised myself. No discoloration. Maybe I had strained a muscle.

"But I paid attention when I noticed a dimple a few days ago," I told the doctor. "That was on the list of danger signals."

The doctor looked grim. "A mass this size is almost certain to be malignant."

His receptionist made an appointment for me to see a surgeon the next Tuesday.

A few minutes later I called Ted from my office in Brock Hall.

"I see," he said, his standard reply when he needs a minute to compose himself.

Next concern. Down the hall to tell Dave, my department chairperson. Supportive as always. "Don't worry about what happens here. Your first responsibility is to take care of this situation. Your life is the most important consideration. The rest of us will take care of your students."

I have a full week to think about all the possibilities before I can see the surgeon.

Tuesday, October 1

A very thorough exam.

The surgeon was positive about everything.

"Yes, surgery Friday," he said. "Yes, probably cancer."

Probably a modified radical mastectomy.

"But then," he said, smiling, "we could be wrong in our expectations. If the mass is not malignant, we'll just remove it, and you'll be back in the classroom on Monday."

He explained the procedure and rationale and gave me nine or 10 booklets to answer questions I hadn't thought of asking.

"I don't feel that we should plan reconstruction," he said. "If this mass is malignant, we'll have to remove so much tissue that the process of reconstructing the breast would be more complicated than . . ." His eyebrows went up as he smiled, meaning, I suppose, to be reassuring, but looking rather helpless instead.

I felt like laughing. Who besides Ted would see my marginally beautiful reconstructed breast? And since he would know it wasn't the real thing, why pretend?

Dr. Greer sent me to outpatient, where I was processed—including X-rays and blood work—so that I could come in Friday morning two hours before surgery was scheduled instead of spending Thursday night in the hospital.

Now I had a new set of booklets to read in order to understand what was happening to me. On Friday I would report to outpatient, where they would prep me for surgery. The doctor would remove a piece of tissue for immediate examination by a pathologist. If the tumor was benign, the doctor would remove just the lump. If it was cancerous, he would remove the whole breast, along with as many lymph nodes as seemed necessary. Malignant tissues would be sent to a lab, where tests would show several things about the kind of cancer we were dealing with. Results would take about three weeks.

"You'll probably need additional treatment after surgery," the surgeon told me.

"How long will I be out of the classroom?"

He lifted an eyebrow. "About a month. You can probably teach during chemotherapy."

I winced at that word.

At home an hour later I called Mom in Montana. She

was already packing for the trip down to spend the winter with us in Tennessee.

"Do you want me to fly down tomorrow?" she asked.

"I'm not dying."

"I don't mean that. Shouldn't I be there with you?"

"You'll be here all winter. That's when I'll really need you." I told her about the chemotherapy.

"You'll lose your hair. You'd better get it cut. And a perm."

"Later," I said. I called the number in Washington State, where Greg and Doug were logging. They wouldn't be back to home base until Friday afternoon. Someone would leave a message for them to call the hospital as soon as they returned.

I drove over to Brock Hall.

"What shall I tell my students?" I asked Dave.

"Major surgery. Outcome uncertain," he suggested. "Tell them that they may have other English professors covering for you from a week to a month, depending . . ."

Wednesday, October 2

Held classes. Explained as Dave suggested.

Took up rough drafts of essays from all classes. Read papers until late. A note tucked in among the papers:

Mrs. Pyke—

  I hope everything turns out OK for you.

 I'll pray for you.

                Love,

                D'Rae

The deeper into the stack of papers I worked, the better I felt. Maybe 20 similar notes were jotted in the margins or at the ends of other rough drafts.

No doubt about it. I have support. Major support.

Thursday, October 3

Up early and read papers almost nonstop all day. On nearly every paper I wrote a good dozen comments. Comments. Are they helpful? Are they even sensible? I probably misspelled hundreds of words in my marginal jottings.

Emily came after supper to spend the night. She made me go to bed early. After she went to bed, I got up for a snack and juice since I can't have either food or drink after midnight, according to the instruction sheet the nurse gave me.

Friday, October 4

Awoke at 3:00. Nobody awake to give me orders. Read the last 10 rough drafts before Emily got up at 5:00.

I dropped the crossword puzzle book and dictionary into my briefcase. Ted carried it and my travel case to the car, and I came with my comp papers to leave for Dave to return to students at 8:00, 9:00, 11:00, and 2:00.

At 11:00 I'll be asleep, unaware of what the surgeon has discovered. By 2:00, I'll know.

We reached the hospital at 8:00.

"Why do you need to be here so early?" Ted wondered, "if everything is already in the computer?"

We started a crossword puzzle. A woman from medical

records came with a readout—to confirm the information. Then a young man—with a name tag confirming that he was a doctor—appeared. He said he was part of the anesthesia team. He asked the same questions his colleague had asked on Tuesday. Then two more young doctors—surgeons or surgeons to be. At any rate with my surgeon's group. Asking more redundant questions.

When they left, Ted grinned. "Practicing medicine?"

"As long as a real doctor holds the knife, they can ask all the questions they want," I said.

"They probably have their forms compared with Dr. Greer's," Ted said, "to see how accurate they are."

"Maybe they're just practicing preoperative bedside manner," I suggested, thinking that while they were older than my comp students, they still had that look about them, aware of their growing professional dignity, but not quite certain how to wear it.

Instead of 10:30, it was 11:30 when an orderly took me to the marshalling area, something totally new to me. Nothing like this in the small hospital where I'd had my tonsils out 40 years ago and later recovered from a car accident. Nothing like this in the little hospital where the children were born.

The gurney driver checked my name on the papers in his hand against the name in black ink on the white board at the station. He wheeled me in and wished me luck.

Then came the man with the IV equipment. Several tries and three nurses later, they finally called one of those nice young anesthesiologists, who threaded a vein successfully and taped the needle with its hook-up securely to the back of my right hand. A nurse snapped in the line from the plastic bags over my head, and I watched the clear fluid moving down the transparent tube into me. Antibiotics, etc.

Dr Greer: "How are you feeling? Any questions?"

The young man monitoring my station began talking to a nurse at the desk about reseeding his lawn. He had sprayed it with herbicide to get rid of weeds. Now he had tilled it and bought fertilizer and grass seed.

"I'll get it replanted during the weekend."

The man at the phone leaned back in his chair. "I don't mean to sound pessimistic. But I did that two years ago. The herbicide got all the living weeds, but weed seeds were not destroyed. I'm still fighting . . ."

"The man at the garden store said he could guarantee . . ."

The nurse at the phone shrugged. "They're selling a product. Of course, it's guaranteed to cure the problem."

I thought about the Johnson's grass in my blueberry patch, which I had sprayed with herbicide. After every rain new spears emerged, but the blueberries suffered even though I had meticulously followed instructions to spray only the undesirables. I saw a sinister similarity between Johnson's grass and cancer.

The clock over the door to the operating area showed 12:00. Someone came for me and trundled my gurney with IV bottles through several doors down the hall.

Lights. People. Action. Dr. Greer, reassuring.

Anesthesiologist: "You'll feel a prick and a sting."

I could hear my heartbeat amplified like the bass drums from a passing car's stereo—only its rhythm more sane. I felt myself dropping heavily through that gulf of sound— falling, fluttering, light, weightless . . .

Chapter 5

THE AWAKENING

I half rouse but keep on drifting.

I have never been so cold—not even when . . .

I'm 22 and walking from my northern Minnesota cabin to the Matelski's farm two miles south. I force one foot to move ahead, then the other. My breath rattles the frozen muffler away from my mouth. Frost covers my eyelashes. My nose no longer drips, because the mucous has frozen in solid plugs, forcing me to breathe through my mouth. When I work the muscles in my face, I feel my nostrils flexing and the hairs inside my nose pulling in the ice. Good, my nose isn't numb. It's still an eighth of a mile from the road to Matelski's house.

Mr. Matelski opens the door.

"Girl, you're crazy!"

I peel off the stiff layers of muffler and try to smile.

"It's 45 below zero."

"So?"

No—not this cold, even then it . . .

I'm wearing four layers of clothes. I'm inside my sleeping bag, under three quilts in my cabin. I tense with the cold, shivering until my stomach and back muscles cramp and my jaws ache. The fire has gone out, and the flat iron between my knees has turned cold. I can't move. Mom always worried I'd freeze to death.

But if this is the onset of death, why the thundering

heartbeat? My whole body jerks with chills. I open my eyes. Twenty minutes to three on the clock straight ahead.

"Why am I so cold?"

"Are you chilly?" She sounds surprised.

Almost instantly other nurses pack heated blankets around me. They talk to me. How do I feel? Still cold? Warmer? Pain? No. In my left arm but not in my breast. No pain at all there.

"It was malignant?" I ask.

"Yes. Pain?"

A little discomfort in my right hand with the IV.

Ten minutes before three.

"Are you warmer now?"

"Comfortable."

Five minutes before three. One by one the nurses remove the four sticky patches from the heart monitor, and the sound of my amplified heartbeat stops. I can barely feel its echo under the tight bandages around my chest.

Ted and Emily are at my room when I arrive on the gurney.

Five-thirty.

Emily has gone to find them some supper, and Ted has gone home for a shower and a change of clothes. I'm tired, but I'm surprised that I don't hurt. A student at the doorway. He comes in with flowers in both hands. He seems confused.

"This isn't intensive care," I tell him. "Come in."

But when I try to talk, I keep slipping out of my own statements into uncertainties and sleep. The student leaves.

Six.

Ted is back with a small brown toy monkey. Emily and I admire it. I reach for it. Just the right size to cup my right hand around so I don't flex the IV needle.

Seven-thirty.

38

I discover when the nurse comes to check me that I have two plastic tubes leading from under the dressing on my chest to two small plastic bottles similar to the squeeze bottles used to squirt ketchup into hot dogs.

"Drainage," the nurse explains. "The fluid is mostly blood now. That's why it's so red and thick. By tomorrow it will be pink, and in two or three more days it will be clear."

Sabbath, October 5

Ted's asleep on the shelf bed under the window, the gray wool blanket gathered around his tucked-up knees. He's been helping me every hour or so all night. He's deaf in one ear. Now he's resting with his good ear down and doesn't hear the nurse come in for vital signs.

"Hungry?" she asks.

"Terribly."

"You'll get a liquid breakfast in a few minutes. Because you're still on IV. The doctor will probably order the IV disconnected before midmorning, and then you'll get a regular breakfast. Real food."

But first the clear fluids.

Ted wakes up. He's brought food from home for his breakfast. He eats dry cereal and a peanut butter sandwich with milk from his Thermos bottle. He hovers. He always does. Now I need his help to get the cup to my mouth. My left arm is supposed to stay on its pillow. The IV limits my movements with my right.

Ted and I study the Sabbath school lesson together and pray. Mostly gratitude today because this much is over, and I still have no pain in my chest. He sits beside me, holding my left hand. I clasp the little brown monkey in my right hand. I've already learned that moving my fingers bobs the IV needle in unnerving ways in the back of that hand. We talk and doze. The tenderest, deepest lovemaking we've ever shared!

About 10:00 the IV comes out. And my real breakfast is hot in the hall waiting. I haven't eaten since Thursday night. I'm not concerned that I'm spoiling my appetite for lunch.

Visitors. College faculty. Friends from Sand Mountain. I'm wrapped in Ted's gray blanket for modesty since I'm not flexible enough to get into a robe.

Emily and our daughter-in-law Martha come to see me. I show them my little "ketchup" bottles pinned to my gown.

Emily shudders. "Do you have to share that?"

Martha, a nursing student, is interested in how much fluid how often.

They leave.

"I can't get used to Emily being an adult," I tell Ted. "Remember how weak she was a year ago with mono? Now she's taking care of me. The world's upside down."

He grinned. "More than once you've complained you've earned a turn to be sick . . . always taking care of the rest of us but never catching anything yourself."

He started to arrange his blanket and pillow on the narrow shelf bed under the window.

"Go home to bed, dear. Go to work tomorrow. I'll sleep through the night. I can get up for the bathroom alone. I'll be all right."

Sunday, October 6

I find my shoes. The nurse says it's all right to walk. In my white surgical stockings — to prevent blood clots — one hospital gown on as usual and another over it backwards, I'm covered, but a strange sight as I stop by the mirror. I've braided my hair myself—with difficulty reaching. I'll walk my two miles in the corridor while I have it all to myself. My lungs feel better in an upright position, and as I walk, even the indoor air feels good surging to the bottom of my lungs. My plastic "ketchup" bottles swing rhythmically under my hospital gown.

Ted's at work today. Will stop to pick me up about 5:30. I watch TV for a while. A medical channel with all the latest info for doctors. Three programs dealing with different kinds of cancer. One suggesting that people with little brown spots like the ones Ted has ought to make body maps with each spot marked so that they can watch to see if any changes occur. I'll have to tell Ted. I worry about him getting skin cancer. Overinformed, I switch channels.

Nothing else catches my attention. I find that the final channel simply focuses on the main hospital hallway leading to the elevators. I turn off the TV, bored. I try to read, but I have a headache.

My surgeon comes by and removes one of the bottles since it has hardly anything in it. He releases me to go home. I dress and gather up my things. Friends from Sand Mountain come and stay until Ted stops by to get me. Even though I walked two miles before breakfast, the nurse pushes me to the car in a wheelchair. Standard regulation.

Dad Pyke calls. He'll be in on the bus tomorrow, coming down from Ted's sister Nytta's in Pennsylvania. In all the excitement we had forgotten he was coming.

Greg and Doug call from Mom's in Polson, Montana. They didn't hear about my surgery because they didn't go back to home base after work Friday but drove straight to Mom's to spend the weekend. They sound awkward.

Worried. Doug has been laid up with two woods-related accidents in the past two years. Greg has been hurt too. But it's different dealing with broken bones than with cancer. The visible enemy is always less scary.

Monday, October 7

Ted leaves for work. I nap.

I wake up. Ann Clark is teaching my 8:00 section. I'm rested now. I ought to get dressed and surprise the kids at 9:00.

I read.

I stand in front of my dresser and look at myself. The dressings are so thick I don't look much lopsided. I unbutton my blouse and look at my "surgical bra," which holds the dressings in place—like an adolescent training bra with a hooks and loops closure in the middle front. Above the dressing, under my left arm, the tissues are puffy. The drainage bottle, which I've pinned to the waistband of my slacks, is half full of an almost clear fluid—like tomato broth today instead of ketchup. Tonight I can take off the dressings and shower.

I empty my little "ketchup" bottle into the marked paper cup and record the amount of drainage and time. I lie down twice and get up. I flex my hand and wonder about the strange feeling, as if something having very long roots has been stripped out from the fingers to the shoulder, something pulled through the incision on my chest. My hand doesn't actually hurt. I don't think lymph nodes have roots like that. I'll have to ask Dr. Greer. I make a very small batch of bread dough. I nap. I read. I make the dough into a pan of rolls and a small loaf of bread. I prepare supper. Ted and his dad come in shortly after 6:00.

"What are you doing running around the house?" Dad Pyke hugs me cautiously with one arm.

"Supper's ready. Wash your hands."

"Are you sure you're up to this much?" Ted asks.

"I'm sick of being in bed. Let's eat."

When I finish, Ted leads me by the arm to the sofa. "You lie down. I'll clean up."

While Ted puts food away and his dad loads the dishwasher, I prop my left arm against the back of the sofa. I wonder if it will eventually swell. Mrs. K must have been about 50 the summer I helped her move into her new house. I think about how horror-struck I was when she took off her loose jacket. Her right arm was huge. During the weeks I worked for her, she spent two hours each afternoon lying on her bed with that arm in a pressure sleeve, forcing the lymphatic fluid back into her body. I imagine the weight of my arm and its bulk—the terrible clothes I would have to make to accommodate an arm of that size. I measure my left wrist with my right hand. My finger just barely reaches my thumb. I'll check each day for changes.

Calls from several family members. Wish good news would travel this fast!

Tuesday, October 8

Tired of doing nothing.

"Want to drive up to Sand Mountain," I ask Dad Pyke.

When we get out of the car, I walk around in the yard for a few minutes and then concede that I'll feel better sitting down. It's just two months since we moved out of this house. I'm not used to seeing my daughter-in-law's sofa and books and clocks in this room.

My grandson Charlie, who is 2½, climbs up on my lap.

"Let me see," he insists. "What did the doctor do to you?"

I draw back my blouse to show him the smooth skin with the pink line and the whiskery black stitches. "The sick part is gone now," I tell him.

"He runs his fingers over the incision, satisfied. "It's all well now," he says.

I hope so.

Chapter 6

PRIMARY SUPPORT

Wednesday, October 9

Dad Pyke leaves with Ted when he goes to work. Will take a bus back to the West Coast. He's 79. In great shape. A card from my 11:00 class. Bruised apple with a thermometer sticking out of it. A full dozen "We miss you"s.

Picked up final drafts of essays from Dave. Began correcting them. Good stuff. Wonderful stuff. Handwritten notes attached to several: "I'm praying for you."

Thursday, October 10

First postoperative checkup with my surgeon, Dr. Greer. He looks at the incision and is pleased. He reads my record of drainage from my bottle. He's glad to see that there's only a tinge of pink, but decides that he'll leave it until next week. With a needle he draws off fluid that has collected in the tissues under my arm and in my side. He presses around the area repeatedly to see if he should try to draw some more.

"Will the fluid just keep building up now? Will you have to . . . ?"

He shakes his head.

"Not for long. A week or two maybe."

"A lady I used to know . . ."

"Not anymore," he assures me. "At least rarely."

"Can I teach one class tomorrow?" I'm not really asking his permission.

"If you don't write on the chalkboard," he relents. "And sit down as much as you need to. But only one class, and if it tires you, tell your boss you'll have to wait longer." He grins. "You must like teaching English better than I liked studying it."

I grip the sides of the examination table. "I can't possibly get well if I can't teach."

"Well," he says, "maybe. In the meantime you need to begin your walking exercises. Stand here beside the wall. I'll show you. Touch your fingers to the wall, and walk them up as far as you can without extreme pain."

I'm surprised that even "walking" my fingers is a little painful. When I get my arm about level with my waist, I'm ready to stop. Dr. Greer notices my expression but leads my arm about four inches higher. "I want you to do this several times a day," he instructs. "We want you to be able to extend your arm straight up with your body flat against the wall."

I watch as he demonstrates, then cringe as he moves me into the desired position.

"Do you have any idea how much this hurts?"

"Not really," he grins. "But I know it's necessary if you want to put that arm back in working order."

Friday, October 11

Ted's day off, so he goes with me to Brock Hall, carrying my briefcase filled with graded essays to return to the group. Students are excited to see me back, thinking that the tumor must have been benign. I explain that it wasn't.

"I feel great," I say. "And I'll feel even better if I can work with you. I can't imagine anything more depressing than lying in bed thinking about cancer. Thanks for your prayers. Now let's just rejoice over what God has already done for me and get on with the business of English."

Ted meets me outside the classroom at the end of the hour.

A card in my Brock mail box from the 11:00 class, the "white space" covered with handwritten notes. Some students do their utmost to sound literary, some are blandly honest:

> *We feel in lack*
> *Until you come back.*
> > *Mike*

> *I know you're going to make it!*
> *Keep up your good spirits.*
> > *Celia*

And similar encouragement from each student.

As we get into the car, I see the laundry all neatly folded in three baskets. Ted has been to the Laundromat facility. Our old washer and dryer wore out before we moved, but we bought a new sofa instead of the appliances. In the coming weeks we may wish we'd been more practical.

Sabbath, October 12

A faculty wife met me on the sidewalk as we left early church to walk across the parking lot to Spaulding Elementary for Open Circle Sabbath School.

"I heard you've been sick," she said.

I took her hand. "No, I haven't been sick. I just had cancer surgery."

She looked puzzled. How could I explain? Would she believe me?

Wonderful to be with friends in Open Circle.

Sunday, October 13

Mrs. Taylor called. She's receptionist in Wright Hall. Answers the main switchboard. She said she had similar surgery nine weeks before mine, and Dr. Greer has asked her to be my support person, giving me information about what to expect. She told me about shopping for wigs and that chemotherapy wasn't nearly so bad as she expected it to be.

Monday, October 14

Nine o'clock class again, then home to rest.

A note from Ann Clark, a colleague in the English Department:

If "Hope is a thing with feathers,"*
Then yours boasts lank wings,
Lifting lilting lyrics
of laughter and love.

Once my daughter Emily sang "You Are the Wind Beneath My Wings" at an academy talent program and dedicated it to me. That was one of the proudest moments of my life—listening to her voice touch each note tenderly, saying those words. Sometimes teens think things like that. They seldom acknowledge that they do.

48

All my life I have been a support person. It feels strange and wonderful to be weak with others supporting me this way. I feel almost giddy, borne up by wings of hope and love and laughter—my friends' wings, my students' wings. And God's wings. I may be "under His wings," but I have a more compelling sense of soaring— soaring with eagles.

Tuesday, October 15

Saw Dr. Greer. He drew off more fluid with a syringe. He pressed around the puffy area under my arm.

"Let's take this thing out," he said, tugging gently on the "ketchup" bottle and its drainage tube. The tube slid like an earthworm from damp soil. It lay in Dr. Greer's rubber glove for a second before he tossed it into the container for blood-contaminated refuse. He lifted my arm higher than felt good. Encouraged me to exercise as much as I could stand in order to restore full mobility before scar tissue prevents it. I did exercises at home. Ouch!

A package came from my lifelong friend Clarene—a small cinnamon bear in a turquoise shopping bag. "I love you" printed on the bag. More support.

Friday, October 18

Jan Haluska, who has been teaching my 11:00 class, came by my office. Did I feel well enough to take back another section of comp? He's facing a pressing deadline for the self-study of the college.

I'm ready. How many naps can I take and still sleep at night?

Sunday, October 20

A woman from the Reach Out for Life group from the American Cancer Society came to the house. She explained about their support group and gave me a bra with a little pocket in one cup and a little pillow to use until I'm ready to order a prosthesis. Several more booklets concerning the services available, advice about dealing with practical problems—emotional problems. She gave me a small rope to run over an open door to exercise my arms up and down and a little red ball to squeeze to strengthen my hand.

As she talked, I scanned the leaflet in my hand, which explained that only women who have experienced mastectomy represent the organization to the new cancer patients. My guest was attractively dressed, poised. I wondered which breast was a prosthesis.

"I hope you can come to our meetings. I think we can help you adjust to the changes," she said.

I hope I didn't sound ungrateful. "I doubt I'll have time to. With papers to correct and student conferences . . ."

She smiled. "If you need us . . ."

---

*Emily Dickinson

Chapter 7

FACING STATISTICS

Monday, October 21

Taught two classes today—8:00 and 11:00. I could feel a physical current of energy each time a student rested a hand on my arm. When I faced the 25 students, I knew they offered me more meaningful support than any organization could.

The 2-year-old daughter of the park ranger where Ted works at Cravens House used to tell her daddy, "Let's go see Teddie."

"Why do you want to see Teddie?" the ranger asked her one day when they had already been over once.

"Teddie woves us," she explained.

My students love me. Nothing feels so wonderful as being loved. If God is love and He has healing in His wings, then human love heals too.

Teaching composition in the computer classroom is fun. Each class period we write more than we expect to. Besides, there are no handwritten materials to read!

Spent a half hour, twice today, exercising. I still have no pain in my chest, but as I began spider-walking my fingers up the kitchen wall after supper, I cried. Ted held my right hand and winced when I hesitated level with my middle blouse button. The pressure of his hand encouraged me to keep going.

I didn't think I could.

But I did.

Until my body was nearly flat against the wall.

Ted handed me a tissue and brought me a chair while I blew my nose.

Tuesday, October 22

Dr. Greer stretched my arm higher. Even though I've been doing my exercises and thought I was doing them right, he found a place where I gritted my teeth.

"I'll give you two weeks to have all the range of motion you'll ever have," he said cheerfully. "What you don't win by then, you'll never regain."

He drew off more fluid with a needle. Not so much this time. He's set me up with a medical oncologist—the doctor who will supervise my chemotherapy.

Wednesday, October 23

Consultation with oncologist, Dr. McCravey. He explains my situation. Reports from the lab that examined my tumor and lymph nodes showed that my cancer was rather rapidly developing and estrogen positive. This means that the tumor is dependent to some degree upon estrogen to support its growth.

Dr. McCravey explains the development of breast cancer. In its earliest form, *carcinoma in situ*, cancer is present in only a small local area and in only a few cells. In Stage I the tumor is less than an inch, with no cancer in surrounding tissue. In Stage II the tumor is between one and two inches and has spread to lymph nodes under the arm.

In Stage III the tumor is larger than two inches and involves lymph nodes beyond the underarm and may be spread to tissues near the breast. Stage IV cancer has appeared in one or more other locations in the body, usually the bones, lungs, liver, or brain.

"In your situation we are dealing with a Stage II cancer," Dr. McCravey says. "If we stopped treatment right now after surgery, your chances of recovery would be about 30 percent. By going with a full series of chemotherapy, we can raise that to about double, and if we add radiation, the chances of recurrence are reduced even more."

He is careful to clarify that the 60 percent plus refers to the percentage of all women who undergo these treatments and that each individual case is unpredictable. "You realize that there is no way to know whether you will be one of those for whom treatment is completely effective or whether you will experience a recurrence in spite of treatment."

I swallow, but the large lump in my throat stays exactly where it was. "I understand."

I will receive three different medications—cyclophosphamide, doxorubicin hydrochloride, and fluorouracil—all injected during the same treatment. There will be six treatments, three weeks apart, beginning almost immediately and ending in late February or early March, depending upon whether my blood count remains high enough to proceed on schedule.

I will experience side effects. However, these are not nearly so serious as they were even four or five years ago. The nausea can be managed quite well by administering a special injection at the time of treatment, and I will receive a prescription for capsules that will help control upsets if they occur when I'm at home. I will lose my hair, but it will come back after treatment ends. I will feel tired and a bit unwell. Mucous membranes throughout my body will be very fragile because they, like the hair follicles, are among the most rapidly reproducing cells and will be attacked by the chemicals meant to destroy cancer cells. My mouth and gums may get sore. My stomach and intestines may become easily upset. My skin may turn dry.

I agree that these side effects are acceptable considering the benefits I will probably receive by going on with treatment. We take care of the paperwork. Dr. McCravey introduces me to Rhonda, the oncology nurse who will administer the chemotherapy.

Rhonda weighs me and tries to find a good vein to draw a blood sample.

"I'm a baby about having blood taken," I confess, feeling silly even mentioning how I feel. "My veins panic whenever a needle pricks my skin. You may have the needle in a good vein, but you probably won't get much blood."

"Hmmm," she says. She tries the needle in several veins before the syringe begins to fill slowly. When she finishes she hands me a cotton ball. "Press that on real firm to keep it from bleeding."

We both burst out laughing. "Sounds like you drilled a real gusher."

She stands back, hands on her hips. "Seriously, you probably ought to have a Port-A-Cath implanted. That way we won't have to go through this each time you come for a treatment. Besides, there's some danger that these chemicals might escape into the tissues in your hand or arm if we don't thread the vein just right. That can be bad. Tissue damage and ugly scars."

"I agree wholeheartedly. Just expecting IVs every three weeks makes me sick."

She sets me up for surgery on the thirtieth.

Dr. McCravey sticks his head through the door. "If you need any dental work, you should get it done this week," he says. "Both chemotherapy and radiation may accelerate tooth decay."

Thursday, October 24

I stop by the beauty school at Eastgate and have my hair cut. The girl stands behind me. Her eyes meet mine in the mirror. She looks scared. I watch as she draws all my long hair back and binds it with a rubber band before cutting it off. She hands me the switch and starts shaping what's left to about three inches everywhere. She begins the perm. Later when the perm comes out, I'm frizzled and fried, which I knew would happen. My scalp burns from all those chemicals.

Friday, October 25

Students look shocked when I walk into class with short hair. A student who comes by my office during the afternoon passes then returns.

"I thought it was someone else sitting at your desk," he says.

"I don't recognize myself in the mirror," I tell him.

Sabbath, October 26

A man in Open Circle touches my arm. "Did you save your hair?"

"Yes."

"I still have my first wife's hair. Her hair was so beautiful. I couldn't look at it for a long time after she died."

Monday, October 28

Dave gives me back the 2:00 section of comp. I make plans to have Port-A-Cath surgery early on Wednesday so that I'll have time to be back at 11:00 for class. Dr. Greer says it takes about a half hour from beginning to end. Should be no problem. Had teeth cleaned since gums will be very tender for several months. One tooth filled during lunch break.

Tuesday, October 29

Erlanger nurse calls to instruct me about surgery. I'm surprised this won't be an in-the-door-and-out-again matter after all. "No food or drink past midnight," she says.

"But I asked for surgery as early as possible . . ."

Evidently arriving at the hospital early does not mean surgery is early or that I'll be leaving within minutes after it's over.

"This is a surgical operation," she says.

"I know, but I have a class at 11:00 and another at 2:00."

"Cancel them."

I hadn't realized that I wouldn't be allowed to drive myself home afterward either. I don't want Ted to take off from work. It all seemed so simple when Rhonda suggested the Port-A-Cath. I feel frazzled. Another tooth filled today. Crown will have to wait until spring.

Mom and Al arrive after 10:00 p.m. Mom calls from Village Market parking lot. She's confused about directions to our house. I run down to meet her, and she follows me home. She's exhausted after driving since early morning, pulling the camper-trailer.

"Sorry," I tell her. "But I'll need you to take me to the hospital early and come back for me in the afternoon."

"We don't have anything else to do," Mom assures me. "We'll just stay by."

Wednesday, October 30

Mom and Al take me to Erlanger at 10:00 for surgery at 11:00. This time I'm awake for surgery, and even though a sheet is placed over my head, I am able to listen in on the activities as Dr. Greer inserts the Port-A-Cath. I return to my room for a brief period and then am dismissed. I'm thirsty, but I have difficulty swallowing ice water. Mom insists that they must take me out to eat since I've had nothing to eat since last night.

Chapter 8

BODY CHEMISTRY

Wednesday, October 30

The Port-A-Cath, according to the booklet Rhonda gave me, is a small appliance that is installed below the collarbone. Just under the skin is a portal with a self-sealing, membrane-covered chamber into which the therapist will insert the special needle for administering chemotherapy medications. Leading from the chamber is a catheter more than four inches long that is inserted into the large vein passing under the collarbone and leading to the superior vena cava. When the therapist inserts the needle, I should feel no pain, since only the skin covers the membrane.

That's what the booklet said. I had no idea how much I would hurt the day after surgery! Opening and closing my mouth hurts. Speaking hurts. Wiggling my middle finger on the right hand is painful. I sit in my recliner with a pile of papers on my lap. I told my students this past Wednesday I would have these back to them Friday, but writing only a few comments on one paper has taken all the grit I have right now. Sorry, kids.

Thursday, October 31

Plugging away. I've corrected papers from one section. I make a small batch of cookies for trick-or-treaters in case they come. Mom makes popcorn and bags it. Only a few children from the immediate neighborhood knock on our door. Others were probably warned by their parents not to bother "the sick lady."

Friday, November 1

I feel like I tried to swallow a rubber bathtub stopper and didn't make it. I don't think I can swallow even water, but it must be nothing more than a sensation because even though it hurts to swallow, the food doesn't stick.

"Please," I tell my students, "don't make me smile. Not even the smallest smile. It hurts terribly, as if the muscles around my mouth are sewn with long stitches directly into the corners of the Port-A-Cath." I turn back all but the three 2:00 papers I didn't finish correcting.

Ted is waiting after class to take me to the clinic for my first chemotherapy treatment. Every time he touches the brakes, I feel like screaming. The Port-A-Cath feels like four pounds of steel sewn into the muscles on my chest. Ted drives very carefully, but we get tangled in a traffic jam on Lee Highway. Sirens ahead, and several police cars maneuver along the shoulders and disappear. Three ambulances, and finally traffic moves enough for us to get off onto another street. We arrive at the clinic too late for my treatment, which, Rhonda says, will take nearly an hour to administer. I'll have to come in next Wednesday. I'm disappointed. I want to get on with this business, yet I hurt so bad I'm almost glad.

Monday, November 4

Back in class with the 8:00 group. Don't know whether Ann Clark or one of the students brought the Snoopy card. A girl on the front row hands it to me. As I look around at their faces, I see they want me to read it now.

It contains 19 handwritten notes around the printed message.

"We're glad you're back."

I want to shout, "Me too!" I'm immensely glad to have all my classes again. No matter how great it's been to have colleagues willing to do my work for me when I couldn't do it, there's no joy like standing here at the front of a classroom with the clock's hands approaching the hour and knowing that for the next 50 minutes the miracle that transfers to my students part of what I understand is going to happen again.

I scan the messages on the card: Assurances of prayers answered and prayers still routinely prayed. A postscript on the bottom of a one sentence note:

Because He lives, we can face tomorrow.
Love and prayers, Kristy

Not so grammatical, but obviously sincere:

I hope you have a soon recuperation.

Tuesday, November 5

Saw my surgeon, Dr. Greer. He thinks the Port-A-Cath incision is healing nicely. I tell him about the lump in my throat. He has no idea why I feel it there.

"We didn't cut anywhere near your esophagus."

I think of Granny Rainey's wax-plugged ears and the fifth-grade health book.

"I know, but . . ."

Somehow, what I think I'm experiencing wants to override what really is.

Wednesday, November 6

First chemotherapy treatment. Rhonda seats me in a blue recliner and encourages me to put my feet up and get comfortable. I take out a stack of in-class writes to read for distraction. She comes with the equipment: a short curved needle with a connective apparatus. She washes the area with several solutions, including one that smells like iodine. She inserts the needle and hooks up the tube to the bag of solution hanging from the stand behind me. She comes with a syringe and inserts its needle into the junction on the line leading from the big bag to my Port-A-Cath. I feel the cold liquid enter the vein in my chest and move down toward my heart.

"This should keep you from feeling nausea," Rhonda explains. She chats as the syringe empties, then withdraws it, changes her rubber gloves, and goes to serve a woman in another chair. The clear fluid in the bag overhead continues to flow. I read a few papers before she comes back with the second medication in a syringe that looks like it holds nearly a pint.

"This one will make your hair fall out," she tells me as the red fluid blends with the IV drip and begins to enter my body. You also need to be prepared for anything at all, because the injections you get today will induce menopause."

That's interesting. One more complication I hadn't thought about.

Two more injections and more information, which is

too much to grasp right now.

"Come back next Wednesday for a blood test," Rhonda tells me as I put on my sweater. "We need to keep close tabs on you so that we know if it's safe to go ahead with treatments. We don't want to let your immune system become so weak that you come down with a bunch of infections. By the way, warn your students not to get too close if they have colds or flu, and be very careful about cuts and scratches. Besides danger of infection, you need to watch out for bleeding since your platelets will be down."

She gives me a small syringe filled with liquid to prevent nausea. "It's so new it's not available except in bulk samples to doctors. If you feel sick, it won't happen for about four hours," she says. "Go home and have a light supper and squirt this medication into a half glass of orange juice before you go to bed."

We stop at the pharmacy for the capsules that are supposed to ward off intense nausea. More than $3 each!

"I don't think I'll need many—maybe eight," I tell the pharmacist.

Thursday, November 7
Dave: "How you feeling after that first treatment?"

Great. No problem. Everything about chemotherapy has been greatly exaggerated.

Friday, November 8
A lot of flu going around. Since he catches flu easily, Ted's getting a shot. Maybe I should if my immune system

is compromised by chemo. I call Rhonda to check.

"Do you usually get a flu shot?"

"No, but then I just never catch the flu."

"Then don't worry about it now. You don't need a shot."

Sabbath, November 9

When I wake up, the house smells strange and bad. Mom smells awful when she comes up to check on me. We go to church in their car. The car smells terrible. The church smells foul, and people in Open Circle Sabbath school, especially those wearing perfume, make everything inside me begin to churn. Mom has a good lunch ready soon after we reach home, but I know before I taste the food that it will not taste like food but like all the things I have been smelling since I got up. I go outdoors to get my breath.

Sunday, November 10

I don't actually feel sick, but smells and tastes are overwhelming. At breakfast I tell Ted, "Even when there's nothing to smell or taste, I keep smelling myself."

"It's all those chemicals," he says, packing the last of his lunch into his bag.

"My urine is dark red. I'm probably sweating the stuff too and breathing out pollution."

"I can't smell a thing," he says as he kisses me next to my ear. "It's just your senses messed up."

Nasty! I correct papers and read to get my mind off it. When Ted comes home from work, we go for a walk. Deep breathing in the fresh air clears my lungs and my brain.

My mouth is a bit sore. I clean my teeth with a cotton swab—as one of those helpful little booklets from the American Cancer Society suggested.

Monday, November 11

Feeling wonderful! Moist cool air outdoors, sweet smelling people in my classes, even those young men with their heady cologne.

Wednesday, November 13

Finger stick blood test. Normal.

"You must be eating right."

"I am."

Mom keeps drowning me in grape juice and has brought me fresh grapes twice during the past week.

Ted and I stop at the supermarket on the way home and indulge our love for fresh vegetables and fruits. Kale, spinach, Swiss chard, collards. Carrots, beets, turnips. Oranges and apples. No grapes.

The inside of my nose and mouth are sensitive—as if the outer tissues have been peeled away, leaving nerves exposed.

Chapter 9

THE BALD HEAD
IN THE MIRROR

Wednesday, November 20

Finger stick. Blood still looking good.

"I don't think I'm going to lose my hair," I told Rhonda. "A friend has loaned me this terrible long black pageboy. I thought she was joking, but . . ."

"Better shop for a nice wig right away so that you'll be prepared," Rhonda chuckled. "Maybe it will take one more treatment, but you'll be bald. Just wait and see."

Thursday, November 21

When I brushed my hair this morning it came out by handfuls. By the end of the day the wastebasket in my bathroom was half filled. Roughly half of my hair. But I still had more than many women do.

My scalp felt dry and itchy. I couldn't help at least touching the itch, and each time I did, another handful of hair. The back of my recliner was covered with hair after I corrected comp papers there this afternoon, and the back of the sofa looked the same when Ted and I finished working our ritual crossword puzzle before going to bed.

"What will I look like in the morning," I wondered.

"Like me," Ted chuckled.

He's been bald for years.

Friday, November 22

Lost as much hair today as I did yesterday. When I reached up to rub an itchy spot during 11:00 o'clock class, my hand came away filled with hair. A student gasped.

"I won't have a chance to shop before Tuesday," I warned. "Be prepared to see me in a wild borrowed wig on Monday." I shuddered, thinking of the black pageboy.

Sabbath, November 23

Bright and warm for this late in November, the breeze felt threatening as it ruffled my thin hair this morning. I have always known why Ted reached for a cap upon leaving the house and why wherever he is that cap rests on his knee or a nearby table.

"Wish I had a hat now," I muttered, thinking of something cozy like the Fat-Hats I bought the kids the winter we went to Montana for Christmas. But not now after I have spent 20 minutes fluffing my hair enough to cover the bare places.

Ted took several pictures after church because Mom asked him to. I guess just in case my hair never comes back.

Monday, November 25

I wore a scarf to school and fluffed my hair in my of-

fice, hoping that my colleague Ann Clark would remember
to bring the wig she promised to lend me.

"It's about your shade of gray and short," she had said.
That sounded better than the black pageboy.

"What's wrong with a stocking cap?" Emily asked on
the phone—she who spends hours fixing *her* hair.
"Everybody who matters knows what's happening to you.
Why worry about it?"

"I'm not worried. I just feel naked."

"Then wear a stocking cap. That cute little blue one
you bought last winter and couldn't get on over your
French braid."

"I thought a cheerful Christmas cap would be nice. A red
one with a green sprig of holly and a white pom-pom on top."

None of my students commented about how I looked at
8:00 or 9:00—we were busy with the papers I gave back to
them. At 10:00 Ann beckoned at my office door. She
handed me a paper bag.

"I have a big mirror in my office."

Maybe it was because I still had a little hair, but this
wig seemed to ride up, almost like a beret, instead of fitting
down over my scalp.

"Isn't it a bit small?" I asked Ann.

"Would it stay on if it were any bigger?"

I tugged it down around my ears, and Ann showed me
how to stick the bows of my glasses through the elastic
loops for extra security.

At 11:00 class and again at 2:00 my students said
nothing about the wig. No one smiled, even though I felt
ridiculous. Almost as ridiculous as I felt the day I got my
hair cut and permed.

Tuesday, November 26

I was bald when I got up. Not a mangy-dog patchwork, but bald except for a few stray white hairs waving like cilia on the surface of a paramecium.

"Well, you look like me now," Ted said when he came to the kitchen to hug me before he shaved. I felt beautiful even when I looked over his shoulder at our reflection in the dark kitchen window, one bald head tucked under the ear of another bald head. He loves me. He loves me.

Wednesday, November 27

"New hairstyle," Rhonda commented when I sat down in my blue recliner at chemotherapy—wearing my mixed silver wig.

Just after she plugged me into the IV, another patient came in wearing a stylish black turban that I knew covered a head looking very much like mine. The woman wore an employee's ID tag with her picture and the Erlanger Hospital logo.

"This is my secretary Pam," she told Rhonda. "She came with me to hold my hand."

I thought she was speaking metaphorically until Pam pulled up a chair beside her recliner and did just that.

"Are you ready?" Rhonda asked, getting out her antiseptic.

"This is the medicine that's supposed to prevent nausea and doesn't." The woman in the turban tried to smile but instead began to cry. Pam's hand tightened even before Rhonda inserted the IV needle.

"I'll bring you more roses," Pam said. "Think about *roses*. Think about *spring*."

The woman sobbed, embarrassed, gripping Pam's hand and holding still while Rhonda hooked up the IV solution in the bag above her shoulder.

That's how I'd be without my Port-A-Cath, I thought. *Only even Rhonda wouldn't have the IV hook-up into a vein in two minutes for me. I'd be mildly hysterical before she found a vein that would thread.*

When Rhonda came back to me, she had the syringe with the red chemical, which she had said was responsible for hair loss. Well, this time all *that* was behind me! One less thing to anticipate.

"Correcting student papers?" she asked as she inserted the needle into the connection along the tube near my elbow.

"No, editing something of my own."

She told me about her vacation to Pennsylvania and the paper she had taken along to finish for her graduate class. "I didn't do a thing with it until I got back," she admitted. "But I stayed up until 1:00 Monday morning and got it ready to turn in that evening. What do you write?"

"Books."

She asked about my books, and I told her that I write Christian stories. "Not preachy, I hope. But people dealing with their problems and admitting that God is involved in their solutions."

"Yes," Rhonda said, pulling out the empty syringe and checking to see that the clear fluid from the bag was flowing again.

I watched her pull off her rubber gloves and reach for another pair as she prepared to help the other woman. "The bottom line in nearly every dilemma we come to has spiritual implications," I said. "I like writing about those implications."

Rhonda tugged to get the right glove over the heel of her hand. "It's good when people can realize that," she said.

When she began the red chemical in the other patient's IV, I left my editing in my lap.

Pam had been chattering for several minutes about teaching her 4-year-old daughter to make cookies. Now with the medication ready, the woman in the turban became tearful again.

"I look like a dog with a bad case of mange," she told Rhonda.

"Think about roses; think about spring," Pam said again, smiling broadly. By now I'd overheard enough of their conversation to know that they were both of them single, facing all of life's battles without the comfort of a husband. *She's got Pam here holding her hand*, I thought, *and that's wonderful.*

Then I thought about how I felt at Ted's response to my question, "What will I look like in the morning?"

And that too had spiritual dimensions.

Chapter 10

NATURAL ENEMIES

Friday, November 15

I preached myself a little sermon after going to bed last night. A dear friend, one of my dearest, had been here for the evening, arriving at a civilized hour—8:30, but after I usually go to bed. I had known she was coming and looked forward to her visit—indeed, I enjoyed her visit—but still needed to quote some Scriptures to myself before going to sleep.

"Great peace have they that love thy law, and nothing shall offend them," says the psalmist (Psalm 119:165).

I guess I'm a little like a cat we used to have. I *am* offended when people condescend to me—even precious friends with my best good at heart.

I suppose at least a score of—yes, again—my dearest friends have come forward with helpful suggestions about alternatives to standard medical treatment for breast cancer, each offering some *natural* remedy or some experimental miracle treatment, again *natural*, that a distant cousin or neighbor's aunt finds is really helping her.

Funny how remedies they invariably suggest are supposed to be more compatible with faith and divine healing than the treatment I have chosen—as if scientific research and testing to determine consistency of results are at odds with a consistent God.

"She's doing fine. She feels better than she has in

years," they all say.

"So? What does that prove?" I want to ask. I felt fine. I wasn't sick. I was working as hard as I have ever worked. And I had a rapidly growing cancer. It didn't hurt. So, does feeling great have anything at all to do with beating the disease? *No!* Not any more than feeling rich and increased with goods, in need of nothing has to do with being free from the sin disease.

They forget that marijuana and opium are *natural* remedies, and sin is about as natural to our fallen condition as you can get.

Now, I'm all for good nutrition and believe that is one area of my illness where I can take control of the situation. Gardener that I am, I have always surfeited and almost become drunken on kale and beets and carrots, potatoes and chard and squash, green beans and peas and corn. And I even enjoy fruits. Not quite as much, but almost.

Ted smiled last evening when my friend mentioned, ever so solicitously, that I ought to eat more carrots — preferably juiced — because they have so much vitamin A. One drawer of the fridge was full of carrots last week, and the two of us have eaten half of them since. Not juiced, but whole in their *natural* or near natural state.

When Ted smiled over her head at me, I had a childish impulse to take her to the refrigerator for a look at all the wholesome stuff crammed in. Now, she's a good cook, and I've enjoyed lots of good meals at her table, but I've almost always felt hungry after everything was served, as if abundance was somehow a sinful perversion.

Thinking like that, smiling over her head like that, I missed part of what she said about a book she'd read. Another cancer patient who had cured herself by eating nothing but raw foods. She had even given up the smallest amounts of dates because she could sense that they were harmful to her. Maybe a totally raw diet would help me too.

I thought cynically about the scientifically proven fact that vegetables in the cabbage family provide a cancer blocking element. For at least 15 years I had made sure our family had one cole vegetable each day. So?

While I was preaching to myself in bed an hour later after she left, I remembered the student last year who cleared some of the fog out of my head with her in-class write.

"Why have you chosen your major?" I asked. "Explain in 50 to 75 words."

"I want to be a teacher," Michelle wrote innocently, "because I like to tell other people what to do. It's fun to correct papers. I like the feeling of authority a red pen gives me."

Probably she admitted to an attitude that is frighteningly true of the whole teaching profession. And for all that Solomon says about a wise person listening to correction, it is no wonder that so few students respond favorably to our pontifical pronouncements.

"Your grammar's bad," we say, as if God wrote the *Harbrace College Handbook*. "Mine's good. Notice that fact."

"Your concept of time and space is laughable. If you only knew as much about the universe as I do, . . ."

"If you only understood the economic crisis as clearly as I do, . . ."

"If you could just grasp the principles governing human behavior as I do, . . ."

"If you would just listen to what I know about healthful living, . . ."

"If you would just let me instruct you about the state of the dead, . . ."

I can't remember what was the last "if only" to attach to

the fuzzy salvages of sleep, but when I woke up this morning, the mortar was solid enough on that foundation to support something I read in 1 Peter 2:1-3: "Wherefore laying aside all malice, and all guile, and envies and all evil speaking, as newborn babes, desire the sincere milk of the word, that ye may grow thereby: If so be ye have tasted that the Lord is gracious."

I've been teaching one thing or another nearly all my life. I've run thousands of red pens dry. I wonder if in the process I have perpetuated Michelle's pedagogy. If my students have bristled and walked away from my wisdom, could it be that I projected my own superiority, forgetting that I am myself in the beginner's class?

This whole idea is rather slippery, and I'm not really sure about its thesis, supports, development, and conclusion. The several analogies slide around and don't quite apply as I consider how logic and structure ought to work together. I do know that it all comes together in the word "grace," which I need myself as I deal with petty offenses and which I need to express more liberally in red ink.

When I started writing for money, I often prayed, "Lord, help the editor to like this piece and buy it." Once in a while I'd get a check, but most of the time I got rejection slips. Was God deaf to my prayers? No. I began to realize that if I wanted editors to like my stuff, I would have to write better: accept correction, study my markets, understand my reader's needs, have something significant to say.

People sign up for my classes thinking, "This woman's a creative writer." They think that I'll give them license to gush and ooze, expressing themselves free from all those constraints that they have come to feel limit their own creative souls. After one or two class periods they begin to see that creative energy, as I see it, demands a kind of discipline they had not imagined, and most of them launch into the struggle toward excellence—before I ever see their efforts. I explain how I write and apply the red ink to my own work and write again—again and again.

Patty turned in a wonderful essay in rough draft—the first paper of the fall semester. I marked it a little—not much—and read it in class. Other students were amazed at the quality of her work. Her partner in peer evaluation effused.

"Oh, Patty, how could you do it? And in first draft too!"

"Eighth draft," Patty corrected her.

Patty believed in my grace, but she also knew that she could pay attention to my instruction and apply the principles. And that's work.

Currently I'm reading my Bible through for the twenty-third entire reading—praying through chapters and books. Accepting the red pen. I'm not saying cancer is punishment for anything. But I'm sure God is using it to improve my spiritual health.

On October 14, 1986, in one of my precancer personal devotions, I realized that in many ways I had been resisting God's discipline. It seemed to me that I needed to give God permission for whatever correction He knew I needed. So I recorded the date in the back of my Bible to mark the beginning of the covenant.

"If You know I need major surgery, go ahead and cut," I told the Lord. "However deeply You need to cut to get rid of the problem, it's all right with me."

I wasn't thinking about cancer or physical surgery when I prayed, but about attitudes that were set in concrete and a mulish disposition. Long before I got to the cancer episode, God started the major surgery I'd authorized. He brought me face-to-face with heartaches that, now when I remember them, make the cancer problem seem insignificant. And He showed me that once He's cut away the threatening tumors from my soul, healing does come.

I should have known better, but I tried to use my cancer experience to develop the Sabbath school lesson I taught in our Open Circle—a mini-demonstration of how God manages sin.

"I didn't blame the surgeon for removing the tumor," I said. "He didn't set out to disfigure my body. I've lost my hair, but I believe the chemotherapy is destroying the free-floating cancer cells throughout my body. My oncologist is not mad at me. He's not trying to rob me of my womanhood. He's trying to save my life. He's making war on the malignancy."

I tried to explain how I felt about the saving intent in God's "wrath." How it's sin He's determined to destroy, not me.

As the group was breaking up after lesson study—I should have expected it—a visitor accosted me.

"I have a video you'll love!" she exclaimed with real missionary zeal.

No, I won't! I thought, trying to manage a polite response while she chattered on about healing cancer with herbs and positive attitudes, etc. Finally one of her friends came and took her away.

I know several cancer patients who have agreed with concerned family members and friends that chemotherapy and radiation—maybe even surgery—are choices off limits to the woman of faith. Unfortunately, most of them are now dead, and the others look like death itself, although they claim they feel they are getting better. Chemotherapy may be a drastic treatment, but cancer, like sin, requires radical measures. For me, to deny that fact shows a lack of respect for my own life and what God wants me to do with it.

(Note: The woman with the video died of cancer nearly a year and a half after this conversation took place.)

Chapter 11

TAKING CARE OF ME

Wednesday, November 27

During the past few weeks, I've received dozens of loving messages from friends who haven't written in years. I don't know whether this is because bad news travels faster than good or whether we believe those we care about need us more in adversity than in good times. My lifelong friend Clarene has been an exception. Through the 30 years since our paths separated, her cards, letters, and small thoughtful gifts have been regular reminders that she cares about me.

In all the distractions of illness, hers and mine, she remembers that today is our silver wedding anniversary. As I open her card and read her eight-page letter, I remember that day 25 years ago when Ted and I plowed knee-deep through snow to gather pine boughs from Clarene's dad's Minnesota woods to decorate the church ourselves. I had ordered red and white football mums, but we wanted the church to smell of pine. Ted joked then that he would warn the preacher that his vows to stick with me through "better or worse" did not apply to living in northern Minnesota. It was 20 below zero that morning, and hardly warmer at 1:00 o'clock when we were married—three miles from my childhood home and one mile from Daddy's grave.

Friday, November 29

Since the rest of the family has to work today, we're celebrating both Thanksgiving and our wedding anniversary tomorrow. All day I cook and rest alternately.

When I go to bed, the taste of old silverware warns me that dinner will be for my guests tomorrow, not for me. I feel, not nauseous, just "yucky" as the kids used to describe so many things.

Last treatment was this way too, but now, since I've been through it before, I'm pretty sure that in two or three days, everything will smell and taste wonderful again. But by then, my family feast will be past.

Greg and Doug are just back from Spokane. We've talked on the phone, but they haven't seen me in my wig. It's been years since they saw me even in short hair. And how does the *mater familia* behave if, while putting the final touches on her Thanksgiving dinner, she becomes violently ill from the distorted food smells? Maybe some other year Emily and Mom can make the feast. This year I'm doing it solo—not because I'm naturally contrary, I tell myself, but because all the "literature" from the American Cancer Society says I should indulge myself, pamper myself. This is the one time in my life, the pamphlets assure me, that the most important thing I can do for others is take care of myself, make things as easy and as pleasant for myself as I can.

Coping's the thing. Managing whatever way I can without worrying too much whether I'm creating problems for other people. Sounds dangerously selfish, but it may be at least partially valid. So I'm ignoring the outcries of my family and cooking up a storm. What better way to do what is best for me?

Of course, it's best for me to plan and shop and

bake—to taste and stir and taste again. What absolute delight, what consummate indulgence!

Sabbath, November 30

When we get home from church, I check the oven. The food looks the way it ought to, crisp and bright, but to me my kitchen smells like the upper hallway of the chemistry building during afternoon labs. No mouth-watering aromas—just bitter, burning, choking smells of experiments gone wrong.

Evacuate the building! Let me out! At least open the doors!

"Emily's here," Ted says as he braces the front door open with his unabridged dictionary.

"Mmmmm!" Emily exclaims, kissing me lightly in her dash to open the oven for a look.

I turn on the heat under the peas and green beans. I am beginning to feel tired, not just of smells, but of being on my feet.

"I'll serve," Ted says. But Martha hands baby Danny to Scott as she comes in the front door. She and Emily have the food in serving bowls before I get settled in my recliner. Ted awards the seats, and Greg asks the blessing. While everyone else heaps up plates and enjoys the mashed potatoes and dressing and accompaniments, Charlie talks Ted into olives off the top of the salad. He eats them swiftly, and I taste a bit of everything before the two of us leave the table, Charlie to play, and I—I want to be near the window with some air.

Even after brushing my teeth, I taste corroded silver plate, but the meal is obviously a success. I am too tired to object when Mom hovers over me.

"No, I didn't overdo."

"I'm too full for pie," Emily says.

"I'm not," Greg says, and Ted brings the whipped topping. He's already loading the dishwasher.

"You go visit with Mama," he tells Emily when she tries to take over.

So she comes to sit on my lap, and I see she's worried about hurting me as she arranges her elbows. Her hair spray and perfume smell nasty, but it's wonderful to hold her.

Chapter 12

DEATH IS OK

Ted and I join the students in front of Wright Hall for the lighting of the Christmas tree. Several days ago I noticed the strings of lights in place on the spruce tree growing in the middle of the concourse. Now the crisp, misty evening reverberates with a male voice bleating carols over the loudspeaker and at least part of the college band playing on Wright Hall steps. After a half hour the lights come on for the first time this year, and the crowd surges to the several tables for hot chocolate and cookies. From now until the week of final exams, we'll be out to some Christmas program or another nearly every night.

When we get home, I wonder if it was sensible to go at all. I'm chilled. I'm terribly tired. And I'm emotionally unprepared for the evil chemical taste that chocolate leaves in my mouth now. I go to bed and think about Christmas without chocolate and whether or not we'll put up a tree at home this year. I page through my memories of all Christmases past.

Once when I was in fourth grade I lost the poem my teacher had cut from a magazine and told me to learn for the Christmas program. I knew there was no use retracing my steps the three miles to the school. A slip of white paper on the snow-packed road was gone forever.

Reaching home, I rushed to the barn where Daddy was

doing chores. "Daddy," I told him while he moved the milking machine from one guernsey to another, "Teacher will be mad. She'll kill me."

"Don't worry," he said. He straightened and hitched up his overalls. "Don't worry. We're poets."

An hour later after supper was cleared from the table, Daddy got out a tablet and a pencil. "Now, tell me about that poem you lost. What was it about?"

"Spruce trees. Christmas trees."

"Fine," he said, settling me in a chair, then sitting down beside me. "We know about trees. Now let's write our poem."

All the lights in our house were out by 8:00 that night because we had to get up early to milk in the morning. But when I went to sleep, I was confident about the Christmas program. Daddy hadn't said so, but I knew he was certain, as I was, that our poem was better than the jingly thing I had lost.

The next day when we practiced at school, I repeated our poem from memory. My teacher didn't notice the substitution. I guessed she had read only the title of her poem when she cut it out of the *Grade Teacher* magazine.

But in that one encounter, Daddy defined me as a poet—I was a poet, just as he was. That was all the affirmation I needed. I have never needed permission from anyone else to be a writer—nor anyone else's approval. In the nearly 40 years I have been trying to sell my product, I have written weakly and badly for many reasons, but when I have written anything good, I have written, not for editors or the readers of their magazines, but for Daddy, my spirit reaffirming things he discovered about what matters and what does not.

Talking with people about my situation, I shift back and

forth between "had cancer" and "have cancer." There's no way of knowing which it is except by continuing to survive.

There isn't even a shade of panic — just a feeling that I might be going to miss something important, like the child sent to bed while everybody else stays up. I always wished Daddy could have seen my children — when they were babies, how he loved babies! — when they were toddlers — on big occasions like baptisms and graduations — and Christmases. But as far as missing something myself, I guess no matter how long a person lives, that feeling is likely to linger, even if it's just to see the next birthday.

I keep thinking about the terribly hot summer of 1980 and that night in September when the first rains came. We were all in bed before 9:00. The phone rang at 11:00. Ted was on the stairs, had the hallway light on before I realized that it was the phone. I listened, wondering who would call us this late.

"I see," he said in an unnatural voice. "Yes, of course. I see."

I knew already that he was listening to bad news. I reached for a housecoat and went to the top of the stairs. He sat on the third step from the bottom, sat the way people sit at funerals.

"I see," he said again and again. "Of course. Yes, of course."

He did not hear me above him, and I sat down to wait. Someone was dead. He had said nothing to indicate it — but only death would explain his formality.

It was his sister Nytta, calling from southern Mexico, I realized. And his mother was dead. I went down to sit beside him on the third step from the bottom, for the first time aware of the rain coursing down the glass on the door.

The telephone conversation went on for more than a

half hour. When Ted hung up, he stood, but his body drooped. "She's gone," he said. "Mother's dead."

"I know."

In any crisis we walk. He got an umbrella before he thought about putting on his pants and shirt.

"No need to tell the kids before morning," he said as I tied my shoes.

Rain streamed down the tractor road between our house and the church. The flashlight's beam darted ahead of us, waiting for us on roots and puddles and other hazards. We came out of the woods into the first field. We skirted the hole dug by truck and tractor tires getting stuck spring after spring where the frost was slow to come out of the shaded earth. The hole was filled with rain and flowing a stream out into the corner of the field now. We came out by the second field, our shoes soaked, walking in rainwater an inch deep in the road. We walked far enough to see the floodlight shining on the church roof, stood for a few minutes, then turned back home. Instead of turning to the house, Ted shone the light further down the field toward the big building he and the boys were constructing.

We climbed its back stairs to the second floor and threaded our way between stacks of lumber in the hallway to the front where windows would be. For hours we sat there, talking sometimes, sometimes silently holding hands.

What do you do when you can't go to a funeral? Nytta had said that their mother must be buried in the morning according to local law. We couldn't even get to Mexico City that soon, let alone Tuxtla and finally Comolapa and Bella Vista. So Nytta and Ted and their brother Dick on a three-way phone call had decided that we should not try to come. Elwin was there for comfort and support. The people at the mission were like family.

So we sat watching the rain slow and stop. We watched the moon come out and mists rise out of the fields and trees. Ted talked about childhood, when his mother was young—many things he had told me repeatedly, others he had never mentioned, dredged up now by grief that reached the bottom layer of his memory. Before dawn we went back to the house to stretch out in our bed and wait another hour to set the day moving.

"I'd rather go to school," Greg said. Doug looked uncertain. Emily bit her lip and nodded.

Friends took over at the day-care center for the elderly which we operated at the time. Ted and I spent the day going through his mother's picture albums, beginning to end, documenting her lifetime in her precise way with dates, names, locations, and occasions. Other albums contained cards she had received for birthdays and graduations since childhood. Letters of appreciation from former students, congratulations on her accomplishments, and one whole book made up by fellow faculty when she retired from the Walla Walla College school of nursing.

The children were solemn when we picked them up from school, grieving themselves, but uncertain how to act and talk on such occasions. They knew how Sand Mountain children were supposed to behave when a grandmother died, because deaths were social situations they had witnessed—the calls on the church's hotline, preparing food for the bereaved family, going to the funeral home, where the family received guests until late at night. The laughter and tears, the family jokes, and sad country music at the funerals. But how were they to behave with their grandmother lying dead 3,000 miles away?

"Everybody at school said we should go to Mexico," Doug said.

"That's stupid," Greg said. "They don't know how far it is. Uncle Elwin can't fly out to get us at the big airport and leave Auntie by herself. Besides, Grandmother is already buried."

"That's what I said," Doug muttered.

"Adam gave me some glitter," Emily said. "Teacher let us two make pictures all day."

A few friends came. We had a memorial service at the church. But without a body to bid farewell, few people came.

Two months later another phone call from Mexico. Elwin, flying some pastors into a remote area for baptisms, had crashed into a mountain. Nytta had not known for sure until she went herself on horseback to the wreckage. With fellow workers, she buried him where he died. Her four children, all in the States, went to her.

I remember Nytta's loss and wonder if Ted is prepared should I die. Most of the time I feel confident. Other times, like today after treatment when I'm bloated with all those deadly infusions, I try to figure out a budget that would allow Ted to manage on one income. He'd either have to find another working wife in a hurry or sell this house and go back to live in our house on Sand Mountain. It's paid for, and he'd be among old friends there.

Chapter 13

Now

A ll my life I've been saving up, putting things away for someday—as if the good things are too precious to use.

When they married during my senior year in college, Mom and Al pooled furniture and tea towels, vacuum cleaners and tablecloths, from two households. Shortly after their wedding Mom was shocked when Al brought out boxes of linens he and his first wife had received as gifts at their wedding 16 years earlier. His wife had thought them too pretty to use—was saving them for special occasions. She died after being married to Al for 12 years, never having taken her loveliest things from their gift boxes.

"I'm going to use everything," I told Ted when we were married. "I'm going to wear out every towel and pillowcase. There won't be a thing left for *your* second wife. She'll have to start out with her own wedding gifts."

We laughed at the time, and through the years we've laughed again and again as I gave Ted thin, faded towels to wash the car. When I broke a goblet or a fruit bowl, I comforted myself that my marriage was more durable than my household treasures—that I was alive and well to use what I had left.

But I've been as foolish a saver as anyone else, in spite of my resolution, saving a favorite blouse or sweater for the most special occasions until it was hopelessly out of style, putting off vacations — or even simple pleasures — because I thought I was too busy to stop the job I was doing. Cancer has changed my perspective.

Probably this change has been most dramatic in my marriage. Both Ted and I realize that this could be our last year together. We've decided to do those things now that we had planned to do later — trips, books, musical programs. We decided that now there is nothing more important than being together. Nehemiah told Sanballat and Geshem: "I am doing a great work, so that I cannot come down" (Neh. 6:3). I'm beginning to feel that way about my marriage — that it is the one great enterprise of my life, and whatever else I might have to leave unfinished if I don't recover, what's between Ted and me will be complete.

Wednesday, December 11

Floyd Greenleaf, our academic dean, asked me a while back to speak to the faculty at the Soup and Crackers Luncheon today. "How to Write a Book." I explained a few things about paying attention to people and things. "Writers write," I told my colleagues. "If you want to be a writer, write. Don't keep talking about it. Do it."

I went to school with a lot of people who had more talent as writers than I had, and there was no doubt about it, they could certainly outspell me. And they could type. Some of them talked about books they were going to write someday. One classmate wrote three drafts of everything from shopping lists to memos to the history professor — the final draft always in Spencerean script. She was sure she would write several best sellers, become rich and famous, and then someone would track down all these memorabilia for some museum. I've never seen her byline, and her name does not appear with brag lines in the alumni newsletter. So much for all the wasted memorabilia!

I'm not exactly famous, but I have doggedly persisted in writing. I'm a writer because instead of dreaming about writing someday, I sit down and do it now.

Basically that's the attitude I'm learning to apply to the rest of my life—I've decided I've got to quit planning to live and start living each day as fully as I can while I have it.

Several years ago a friend gave Ted four lovely oil paintings. We hesitated to spend the money to have them restretched and framed. We've decided to do it now—to get them up on the wall where we can see them. Now.

When we moved into this house we loved the yard with its wonderful oaks and tulip poplars. We liked the inside too except that we got almost no sunshine in the living room or my study. And everything except the kitchen and our bedroom, which were wallpapered, was painted the color of Dijon mustard, an exact match for the smell that swamped me after chemo treatments! When we moved in during August, we decided we would have to wait a year before spending money on paint since it was a careful paint job and looked quite new.

Last week Ted made a decision. "We'll paint now."

After Sabbath we went to Wal-Mart to get supplies and ended up buying a large potted dwarf shefflera. Ted's a fussy painter, so it took him several days to paint the living room and hallway. The results were bright and satisfying, a color called Silver Thread, which is like reflections of winter sunlight on snow. And then we hung the lace-trimmed curtain Mom bought in Norway years ago. I'm becoming giddy with the idea of change.

90

For most of my life I didn't have time for any activity unless it put food on the table or clothes in the closet. For the first time in my life I'm learning to play with a clear conscience. Ted brought me a jigsaw puzzle of the German Alps. Very difficult. I've spread it out on the dining room table, and I intend to take time for the pleasure of putting it together. This week.

Wednesday, December 25

Doug and Emily come. Our first year without the whole family together. Open gifts together while dinner finishes. Immense teddy bear slippers from Emily. A blender from Doug. Books and other sweet important things from Ted. We're giving each other a trip to Washington's art galleries for Christmas. Almost too tired to sit up after dinner. The kids leave about 4:00, and I go to bed.

Friday, December 27

At 2:30 both Ted and I were awake to stay. I packed our lunch, and Ted put our bags in the car. We left home at 3:00. Visited Clarene and her husband, David, in Richmond on Sabbath. We stopped to see Civil War battlefields at Wilderness, Chancellorsville, Spotsylvania Courthouse, and Fredericksburg. It was beginning to rain as we reached the top of the hill overlooking the Rappahannock River. Checked into a motel. Exhausted. Glad Ted called a halt about halfway on the walking at those battlefields.

Monday, December 30

Left Fredericksburg at 7:00. Ate breakfast on the way to Washington. Reached Mall at 9:00. Parked at Washington Memorial and walked through Mall to old Smithsonian building. Enjoyed statuary. Walked on to Capitol. Ted took pictures of paintings in rotunda. Down to National Conservatory to see poinsettia show. To National Museum of Art—17th and 18th century British and American. Lunch. Ted moved car. Left me at Museum of American History. Jewish group performing thirties' Yiddish music on first floor. When Ted returned we toured "America After the Revolution" home displays. Briefly to Museum of Natural History. About 5:30 to our bed and breakfast in Takoma Park.

Tuesday, December 31

Waffle breakfast. Took city bus to Metro station. Took train downtown. Walked to National Museum of Art—East. Waited in line for tickets to Circa 1492 exhibit and went in directly, although there were hundreds of people waiting. Crowds packing door area, but we could take our time looking once we were inside. Began in Europe, showing cultural and scientific atmosphere of the times then moved on around the globe to show the world as it was on the eve of the discovery of America. Africa. Asia. Central America. South America. Two marble figures from Ettowa Mounds near Atlanta. Wondered what was the condition of the heart for those Native Americans circa 1492 who shaped that man and woman from stone and buried them. Small French Impressionist display as we came out of 1492. Delighted by the hundreds of small canvases with their details of the human faces and water and flowers and homes in colors that got a hold on my vitals, and produced visceral responses. I want to reproduce colors like that on a flat sheet of paper in my books—to force my reader's imagination to reproduce human realities and grow wise.

Ate snacks from our pockets and then returned to American Museum of Art—West to see French Impressionists and Dutch Masters, often sitting absorbing the mood of a single painting for 20 or more minutes. Took Metro back to bus station. Had excellent Chinese food where we got off bus. Walked to bed and breakfast. Watched TV, including Berlin Celebration with Beethoven's Ninth Symphony. I knew the German choir was singing different words, but I was singing the words:

"Joyful, joyful, we adore Thee,
God of glory, Lord of Love . . ."

So very tired, but comfortable and satisfied. My stamina might be diminished from normal, but I still feel pretty good for a cancer patient. Ted has been careful to match his pace to what I can manage.

Chapter 14

BECOMING A SURVIVOR

Thursday, December 19

Note from Kim Walters:

I'm sorry to hear about your operation. I know it wasn't easy, and my heart goes out to you. It may help to know that my uncle was diagnosed with cancer this summer and was completely healed because of all the prayers. Your name was mentioned at prayer meeting, and my brother's Bible study group is praying for you. Your creative writing class was my favorite in four years of college, and I think you're a wonderful teacher. After talking with you on Friday evening, I couldn't let this week go by without letting you know I care. I'll be praying for you.

Monday, December 23

This has been a rough weekend, I feel guilty even saying that when I realize what "rough" means for some people. But rough for me. I've felt tired and nasty since Friday morning—evil smells, vile tastes. I open my mouth and taste the world like a choking mouthful of paste. I don't want to sense the world around me like that—constantly railing about what isn't right.

We've opened the windows and doors, because it's only our own human smells that are offensive—our cooking and breathing smells, our soaps and deodorants and coverup. It's raining—mild, dripping, and wonderfully clean outdoors, and letting that clean into the house helps.

Sabbath, January 4

To early church for Communion. Ken Rogers spoke about asking Jesus to come into our lives and settle in. Ted and I participated in family footwashing. Rested after spaghetti and vegetables for lunch. Read.

Sunday, January 5

Read Genesis 9-11, Psalms 4-6, Joel 1-3, and Proverbs 30. One chapter suggested another. Baked bread and began cleaning my study while Ted washed clothes. Worked sorting manuscripts, etc. nearly all day. Mom and Al came back from Nashville about 3:00. Had been visiting Aunt Anne and Corky.

Thursday, January 9

I'm halfway through my chemotherapy. Third treatment yesterday. The woman who came in at the same time asked me how I was feeling.

"Great," I said.

"Me too," she said. "Praise the Lord!"

She was finished with the treatment before I had my coat off.

"Daily injections all this week," she explained. "But I have a Port-A-Cath too, and it's not much trouble except for the time it takes to come in."

My IV wouldn't flow. Rhonda flexed the lines and my arm, but nothing happened.

"Better send you next door for an X-ray to see if the tube in your vein is in position," she said.

Next door meant Parkridge Hospital—not Erlanger, where I am a regular patient. Here I went through outpatient and then to X-ray. An hour later I was back with Rhonda. No problem with the Port-A-Cath tube, so we tried again. At first no movement, then as Rhonda put my recliner back and drew my arm down almost to my knee, it started. Great!

Wednesday, February 19

Last treatment. IV flowed without all the fuss we've had the past four times. Relief!

Walking two miles daily now—probably why I feel so much less nausea than other times. Still feel like I have a big plug in my throat. Weak.

Tuesday, February 25

Took one of those $3.00 capsules that are supposed to knock nausea.

Wednesday, February 26

Misty early morning walk. Turned colder all day. Blood machine down at clinic. Did not have blood test today. Napped at noon. Took tax materials to be processed.

Nausea yesterday—all day. Took another capsule since I paid for eight and still had six left. If it helped, I'm glad I took it, because even after the capsule I felt rotten. Who knows how it would have been otherwise. Classes—sort of. My students are wonderful. This morning a lump in my throat so tightly fixed I could hardly swallow water at 5:00. It's relaxing a little. Home at 5:00 p.m. To bed at 7:00.

Thursday, March 5

Breakfast on the deck. Planted Mom's red dogwood. She and I went shopping at Hamilton Place. She bought shoes, dress, and blouse. We ate lunch at Morrison's. I bought a bale of peat, a small cedar, and two tomato plants. Rain beginning as we came home. Light rain during evening. Walked three miles.

I think my eyeballs were sunburned during vacation while I worked without sunglasses. Since I have no eyelashes or eyebrows, my eyes are exposed to much more sunlight than otherwise. Also have problems with fine dust and large particles getting in my eyes.

Chapter 15

RADIATION

Wednesday, January 22

Saw Dr. Davidson at 9:30. Now, here's a woman I can trust! She's about my age and as substantially built as I am. She even has graying hair in a single braid down her back. Very sensible! Very trustworthy! I can see she shares many of my values, which are, of course, not just superior but correct. I can imagine Emily voicing my reactions.

Dr. Davidson explains the treatments. There will be 29 sessions with radiation. Five days a week for five and half weeks if my skin can take it. While chemo was initiated almost immediately after surgery in order to destroy any free-floating cancer cells that might have escaped through the lymphatic system and taken root in other body tissues, radiation will be directed specifically into the tissues of my chest, where cancer cells might be embedded in bone or other tissues unaffected by the chemotherapy.

"Recurrence of breast cancer is most likely to be in the lungs or in bones of the chest," Dr. Davidson tells me.

"What kind of damage can I expect?"

She raises an eyebrow. "We have much greater control over the depth and strength of radiation than you would imagine. If we're to reach to the inner surfaces of your ribs, we cannot avoid touching the outer surface of your left lung." She taps my chest to indicate the spot. "But since you're a heavy walker and have never smoked or even lived or worked with smokers, your lung capacity is great enough that you shouldn't notice a loss. You *will* get a good suntan on the area treated, maybe even a mild burn."

"How about my energy level?"

Dr. Davidson grins. "Most of my patients who have never had chemo think that radiation really zaps their strength, but people like you, who have been used to feeling tired and weak from chemo, generally experience an increase in energy. You'll probably start feeling better right away."

She tells me that I'll come in each day at a designated time, will walk into the treatment area when my name is called, will lie down, get up, and walk out—all in about 15 minutes. The daily drive will take nearly two hours, counting both ways. I wonder how long it will take me to find a parking place.

We set up an appointment to begin in mid-March.

Monday, March 9

In for radiation set-up at 9:30.

"This may take as much as two hours," Dr. Davidson told me in January when we set up today's appointment. So I came with a briefcase full of papers to correct during the waits. But there were few, and those short.

Dr. Davidson came in first to locate strategic points on my chest. She used a felt marker. When she finished drawing red and green lines, I felt like a map. A team of technicians took a series of photos and X-rays to be used in creating some kind of template through which radiation will be directed to exact locations, while the plate protects other areas from exposure.

Back to my office for student conferences and faculty senate during the afternoon. Planted three raspberry bushes in a hurry before leaving for the travelogue *Wild Rivers U.S. and U.S.S.R.* Closed my eyes during much of the program because they hurt.

Wednesday, March 11

First radiation treatment. A nurse led me to a wall of storage cubes.

"This is your gown," she said, pulling one out of a box marked PYKE. "Put it back here each time after you have a treatment."

She showed me to a dressing cubicle next to the door marked TREATMENT ROOM — DO NOT ENTER.

"Remove everything above the waist and put on the gown with the opening in the back," she instructed me.

"Mrs. Pyke?" called a voice from outside the curtain. "We're ready for you."

I followed two young women through the door, around a corner, into a room dominated by a large treatment table and a monster machine swinging on a arm over the table. One woman set a step stool for me and helped me climb up and lie down.

"Put your left arm back here," said the technician who said her name was Connie. She strapped my arm with a hooks-and-loops fabric to a very cold arm rest.

"Now your right arm over here."

They chunked the new templates into the machine and lined me up so that the map on my body matched the marks projected through some kind of transparency and onto my skin.

No one was touching the light switches—not that I could see, but the lights kept coming on and going off in the most disconcerting way. A beam of red light crossed just over my body to a mark on the opposite wall. The room was cold. I was glad they had not asked me to take off my shoes. I kept waiting for something to happen, but although the two women kept going and coming, I heard nothing indicating that the machine had come on.

There was nothing the matter with the machine dispensing radiation, the technicians assured me, but the table's power connections were messed up, and they had a lot of trouble getting me into exactly the position necessary.

Finally they explained that I would have to wait until an engineer took care of the problem. A half hour later, still shivering in my thin cotton gown, I was relieved when the machine above me buzzed briefly.

The technicians returned, and while the other woman readjusted the machine's head above me, Connie patted my chest with her cold hand.

"This will feel chilly," she warned me the instant she slapped a heavy pad over part of my chest. It felt like something fresh out of the freezer. Connie and her friend disappeared in the dim light, and the machine buzzed again. I counted to 90. The buzz stopped. They got me in four positions before pulling off the straps.

"Stop at the desk for tomorrow's treatment time," Connie said as she helped me off the table. "Tomorrow it really will take only 15 minutes. Promise."

The receptionist stamped my parking ticket.

"We'll be ready for you at 9:15."

So late that I went directly home for an early lunch, then back to office to correct papers.

Tuesday, March 24
Up at 5:00. Treatment at 8:30. Dr. Davidson remapped me for the second half of treatments. Technicians pricked me with five tattoos the size of a blackhead to mark the corners of treatment areas in case other radiation is needed if cancer comes back. Finger stick blood test.

Friday, March 27
First day with new setup. Dr. Davidson supervised. Out at 10:00.

Tuesday, March 31
Radiology called. The treatment table is down. Treatment to be at noon on the other machine. Called again at 12:15. Dr. Davidson said no treatment today.

Wednesday, April 1
Up at 5:00. Don't know when treatment is scheduled. 8:30. Chest is beginning to turn pink. Chin itches. Behind left ear too. Trouble swallowing becomes more severe each day, but eyes improving. Collected odds and ends of a little package for Charlie to open while traveling—coloring book and crayons, preschool scissors, self-sticking paper loops, stickers and books to put them in.

Friday, April 3

Treatment at 8:30. Saw Dr. Davidson. She says skin is not as pink as usual for patients at this point, so I will probably be able to tolerate the full 29 treatments.

Sabbath, April 4

Before church walked three miles on the ridge. Dave Smith had Sabbath school lesson. Elder Kulakov had sermon. Home at 11:30. Walked one mile loop before preparing dinner. Greg and Martha and the boys came over from Sand Mountain for dinner. After the meal I was washing Charlie's face in the bathroom. He noticed the red marks showing above my blouse.

"Grandma, do you have an owie?"

"No, that's just a felt marker," I reassured him.

He looked puzzled and then accusative. "*My* mommy won't let me mark on my belly with markers."

Sunday, April 12

Radiation is nearly over. Six more treatments, to be exact, unless I blister badly. In that case, we'll stop on Wednesday. Today I have only a small patch of blisters in my arm pit at the very corner of the treated area. My chest is a strong pink within the red, black, and green marked blocks.

Dogwoods have opened the past two or three warm days—azaleas too on the hill behind the house.

Wednesday, April 15

Treatment at 8:30. Saw Dr. Davidson and had blood test. Weighed more than I would like anyone to know, even though down two pounds from two weeks ago!

Monday, April 20

Last treatment at 8:15! Saw Dr. Davidson.

Wednesday, April 22

Radiation area very sore and weepy. Had to apply ointment Dr. Davidson gave me and bandage the area. Planted azaleas by Mom's pink dogwood in the backyard. Corrected CW papers until bedtime.

Thursday, April 23

Napped. Lots of pain with radiation burns.

Wednesday, May 20

Went with Ted to work. Walked Cravens Terrace then trail to the Civil War Rifle Pits and back to Cravens House. Then to Dr. Davidson's office at Erlanger Radiation. She is pleased with condition of my skin and with my general well-being. I asked her my list of questions.

1. Has the soreness I've felt in area of upper ribs and clavicle since radiation been a normal result? **Yes.**

2. Is the small scaly patch on my throat dangerous? **No. Probably a blemish dried up by radiation.**

3. Is it all right for me to start a diet to take off the pounds I gained during treatment? **Yes. A sensible diet. No less than 1,200 calories a day, and no greater than one pound per week weight loss.**

4. Is it safe for me to be exposed to sunlight? A friend said I shouldn't get out in the sun at all now. **No sunbathing, of course.** (She disapproves of all sunbathing for anyone. It's a high-risk activity. But normal sun from moderate outdoor activities is fine.)

5. What can I do about hot flashes? **No hormones. Try vitamin E. Some researchers report it helps. But it might not.**

6. How often should I come in for mammograms? **Annually.**

Dr. Davidson wants to see me every six months.

Chapter 16

THE STUDENTS I LIVE FOR

Monday, January 6

My reader, Michelle, had syllabi and other handouts ready, so today I had only to lay out the materials for this week's classes and review my beginning-of-the-semester lectures.

Jim, who was my student five years ago, came in to visit for more than an hour. Larry, who will be my student this semester, brought me a recent research paper so that I can judge whether creative writing will help him become a better historian. I gave him a copy of my rationale for the class.

I've mentioned this to several of my colleagues during the past months, and Ted and I have talked about it repeatedly. There is something wonderful going on among my students this year. Something difficult to define. A few weeks ago a girl who didn't seem particularly spiritual come into my office and closed the door behind her. She sat down beside me and reached for my hand. I was expecting her to beg for mercy about a late paper or to help her out of a sticky personal problem. Instead, she gripped my hand between both of hers, bowed her head, and began to pray for me. She obviously was talking to Someone she knew very well and trusted, and when she finished, I felt an unprofessional unconcern about her dark red nails and the earrings that swung through her masses of dark curls when she bowed her head.

Often these past three months I have felt as if my students had all of them talked my situation over and decided to carry me through this school year in their arms. I've felt their physical vitality pouring into my body when they hugged me. I've felt able to manage on days when I knew my teaching lacked sparkle, because they kept affirming me, telling me they appreciated my work. I've felt the power resulting from their intercessory prayers, some here in my office and other prayers reported to me in notes and conversations. I've had my own private cheering section, and when I have felt as if I didn't have enough energy to make it through the day, they have been there in the bleachers applauding and cheering when I stumbled around the track. Speaking metaphorically, of course.

God has been using a lot of people to encourage me. But what He's been doing for me through my students is more than wonderful. Stopped by my office on my way to chemo treatment at 9:00. I've reserved Wednesday mornings for medical appointments this semester. Kept my mind off the infusions of chemicals today by studying Comp 102 lecture notes. Classes met at 2:00 and 3:30 Monday and Wednesday.

For years I've used this assignment as an icebreaker in this class, and each year I've written along with the students, but this year it won't be a perfunctory exercise.

"Let's imagine," I tell my students, "that you have died, struck by a speeding car or some swift disease. I want you to write your own obituary. Give the usual information about place of birth, education, and surviving family members, but concentrate on relating your accomplishments that friends will remember with the greatest pride."

Today, as usual, a few students don't know what an obituary is—have never been to a funeral—and many of them seem to think they're immortal. I assure them that writing this in-class essay won't bring about their death any more than writing a will precipitates death for their parents or grandparents.

Now I set about writing my own obituary. What do I want people to remember about me?

I am the daughter of my father and mother.

I am Ted's wife.

I am Greg, Doug, and Emily's mother.

I am Charlie's grandmother.

By the grace of God, I am His child, a teacher and a writer. Everything about me worth remembering demands explanation in terms of relationships and processes. I try to forge a one-page summary of my life.

Primed myself for first creative writing class from 8:00-12:00. Two sections this year at 2:00 and 3:30 Tuesdays and Thursdays with a total of 24 students. We're meeting at tables arranged in a hollow square so that we can look each other in the eye during workshop. I'm excited about the talent present in these groups.

Tuesday, February 4

Ted's into one of those congestions that sometime bring him on the verge of pneumonia.

Spent the morning talking with Eric about *Legacy,* our Writer's Club literary publication. He told me about his plan to write a 40- to 50-page play for his creative writing project.

In inter-campus mail:

I've been praying for you and hearing about your courage and stamina. I'm so glad I know you. You've made me proud, and I pray that others will be as blessed by you as I have been.

Kristin

Friday, February 14

Ted's little better. I went to office until noon. Found long-stemmed rose and card on my desk.

We would like to thank you for your thoughtfulness and your consideration. Your kindness and caring mean a lot to us. Thank you for keeping us in your thoughts.

Love,

Greg and Shawn

Went to vespers. Elder C. D. Brooks of Breath of Life. His sermon on Shadrach, Meshach, and Abednego. "Stand." Hundreds of students stood in response when he asked us to take a position and maintain it regardless of opposition. I couldn't stretch enough to stand as tall as I felt like standing after that sermon! I could see students all around me who were moved as I was. Chemotherapy is one kind of infusion—one that's effective because it kills. This sermon was an infusion of *life*.

I'm chugging away, going to classes, correcting papers, doing all the committee work, but some days when I drive into the yard at 5:15, Ted comes and opens the door and takes my briefcase, not just because he's a very polite man, but because I don't have the grit to get out of the car by myself. This note came just when I needed it:

Dear Mrs. Pyke,

I've been meaning to drop you a note since last week because you looked so tired in the faculty senate meeting. Jeff is a close friend of mine; he's told me about the hard time you're having this year, and I was so sorry to hear about it. I'm keeping you in my prayers.

So many times we take our teachers for granted. I know it's been three years since I took comp from you, but I wanted you to know how much I appreciated your class and your taking time to talk to us individually—not only about the assignment, but also just trying to get to know us a little better. I gained a great deal of respect for you during that class. Jeff always speaks very highly of you. Thank you for going beyond your job description, even when there have been times, I'm sure, you didn't feel like it. It will always be appreciated and remembered more than you know.

I hope that the school year and the summer go better for you. I will continue to pray for you and your family.

Sincerely,

Melissa

To vespers for Southern Singers Home Show. Very proud of Sheldon's performance in "Sinner, Sit Down." I could tell he meant it when he responded to the voice of God telling him to sit down—"My soul's so happy that I can't sit down."

Monday, April 27

Talked with several CW students about their plans to use writing skills in their professions—a couple of historians and a lawyer someday. Have corrected almost all the CW materials now. Late 102 research paper about finished. Urged students to hurry to get in their final assignments.

Not feeling well. While radiation burns are not very painful, they are wearing me down. Cold and windy today. Dogwood winter, which here in the Southern Appalachians comes after first spring and is followed by more spring, then blackberry winter, and finally real spring, which rushes headlong into summer.

Wednesday, April 29

At office 8:30-4:30. Corrected late 102 work and CW tests. Many students came by to talk and say goodbye. One girl, who was my student in grades 10-12 on Sand Mountain and in CW here a year ago, spent a good while talking with me about her future.

A tiny box of expensive chocolates and a note from a student:

Mrs. Pyke,

I wanted to let you know just how much I appreciate all you have done for me this year. You may not realize it, but you have seriously been an inspiration to me. Thanks for all your time and patience! I know my grades probably don't show it, but I learned a lot between the first day of class last fall and now.

May God be with you always. I know He's been looking out for you!

With much sincerity,
Celia

Appropriating the words of Thoreau, this is where I lived this year and what I lived for.

Chapter 17

WATCHING THINGS LIVE

I noticed the way Mom and Ted looked at each other when I started filling a nursery flat with potting soil in mid-January. I knew as well as they did that planting leftover seeds this early was senseless, but I felt compelled to get something new growing. Because there was no window in the house that got enough hours of sunshine for seedlings to flourish, I carried the flat from room to room, settling it at bedtime under the fluorescent light above the kitchen sink. On cold January nights I revised my seed orders and finally mailed them off.

Ted and I made two raised beds in the back yard. I was amazed that after weeks of being waited on I could still carry a five-gallon bucket of soil in each hand. I guess I kept up my strength carrying my briefcase full of Harbrace folders.

I'm dreaming my flower beds into full bloom and my raised beds luxuriant with beets and carrots, lettuce and cabbages. My dreams were heavily indebted to Burpee and Parks seed catalogues, but then, I have 25 years of other gardens to remember, some of them nearly as pretty as the pictures.

Vegetables are so real, so real in their palpability. Not even flowers can be more beautiful than tomatoes and eggplant and crooked-neck squash. And all the wonderful folds and shadows in a leaf of Swiss chard! I'm dreaming.

Friday, February 7

Went to Sand Mountain to get plants. Martha says they will move to Washington State in late March or early April. Charlie went out with me to dig plants. Got Juneberry, fig, Easter lily, pinks, sweet William, bleeding heart, yarrow. Home at 3:30.

Thursday, February 13

Got azalea at Red Food for Mom for Valentine. Ted's still sick.

I thought I might be catching whatever he had, but flooded myself with liquids for several days and thought about spring and roses. I opened my office window and absorbed the sound of gentle rain. Did not catch whatever the bug was, but the chemo treatment was another matter.

Thursday, February 20

Worked on CW papers. Feeling rather bad. Ate very little. Home at 5:00 to bed.

Friday, February 21

Worked at office, correcting last 102 papers and some creative writing. Home for lunch, feeling puffy and rotten. Took nap. Sat most of the afternoon in the sun on the front steps, warming my mind into a half-dreaming quiet as I watched the neighborhood children and dogs.

Sunday, February 23

When I awoke at 2:30, rain provided easy-listening music, playing so low that I rolled over in bed and hummed through another dream. Up at 3:00 to read for an hour— three chapters in Luke. Four psalms. Back to bed to listen to louder rain—my window open. After several naps, awake at 7:00.

I had promised myself two accomplishments for the day—to settle the eight strawberry plants in their new bed and to organize my study. After breakfast Ted read to me for a while. Luxury! We talked about the strawberry bed. Since rain had stopped, we went out and built a low retaining wall and filled dirt behind it.

At 12:00, with precious little done in my study, we went to the garden store for a bale of peat. I allowed myself to be enticed by four primroses. They will be beautiful at the street end of the strawberry bed.

Planted my strawberries near the street and then two eight-foot rows of beets in the raised bed Ted made a month ago.

Tuesday, February 25

It's raining in the background again this 3:30 a.m. I lie in bed, replaying the conversation with Rosemary and Mrs. Gearhart in my office yesterday. Rosemary: "He really believes that everyone can achieve what *he* has—that kind of excellence—in their own fields, of course."

Both Rosemary and Mrs. G. are outstanding teachers, examples themselves of excellence, but they've seen a lot of students fail, and I guess they think that for some people real success is beyond reach.

I'm wondering now as I listen to the pattering rain what constitutes excellence. This looks like the beginning of the generic freshman definition paper on success, with the dictionary quote up front, followed by the many "false but possible" examples and finally the real thing, "my true" definition.

But I wonder if excellence has to move in tandem with prominence. I'm not sure it does any more than the perfection of raspberry red veining the interior of a November acorn and the turgid power of its white embryonic root. Every one of the thousands of acorns underfoot on the Biology Trail on White Oak Mountain has the potential to become a tree, given enough time. All of them won't, of course. And not for the same reasons that people don't always reach their potential. Most of them will be washed like so many pebbles by winter's rains down the slopes into masses of compost. But inside each one is a flush of raspberry red beautiful enough to inspire a sonata.

God planned perfection in small things — grass blades the cattle eat without noticing. The onion on my cutting board, sautéed with no notice of its beauty. Flavor, yes. Recognition and even acclaim are not equal to excellence. I think it is only the human spirit of scrambling up to be noticed that demands that definition.

Of course, thoughtful people notice things. Poets do and artists and musicians — and mothers hesitating for an instant over onion rings before dropping them into the skillet.

Thoughtful people appreciate excellence in other people. But public notice — probably not — at least for most kinds of outstanding performance.

Wednesday, March 4

Cleaned honeysuckle from corner of the backyard. Ted helped me burn the pile of vines and brush. Replanted the birch I brought from Minnesota five years ago and had planted on Sand Mountain.

Friday, March 6

Spaded along driveway and planted the geraniums I kept alive all winter in the garage. Hope they don't freeze.

Sunday, March 8

Bright sunshine in the 80s. Ted and I planted cedar. Bought two peach trees, two apple, and one pear at Wal-Mart. Planted them beside the driveway. Plums on the up-hill side of the house are in full bloom. Hyacinths and forsythia in bloom. Ted helped me plant peony, weigela, and small perennials, including Pink Panda strawberries.

Wednesday, March 11

To family night at the church. After devotional period, we attended a gardening class with "Boots" Kuhlman. Cold with frost. Oh-oh! My geraniums!

Tuesday, March 24

Home at 5:00. Planted two rose bushes in front of house.

Sunday, April 5
Planted carrots and lettuce on my first little terrace. Got peat, an Easter lily, and seven more 89¢ azaleas. Got begonias to set out where the geraniums froze. Ted helped me plant after supper.

Friday, April 24
Corrected CW papers at home until 9:00. In office until 12:00. Home for lunch and corrected some more. All the creative writing papers are in now! To garden store for annuals—impatiens, petunias, pinks, sweet Williams, candytuft, tomatoes, and peppers. At home Ted mowed lawn and I corrected papers.

I've finished this school year! After turning in my grades, I took a bucket of old fashioned iris to Mrs. Gearhart. She insisted I sit down and have some of her cornbread baked in a skillet—wonderful with milk! Then we went outdoors to admire her yard and garden. When I got home I tried to start the weed trimmer but gave up. Instead I pulled my first radish, washed it under the outdoor faucet, and sat on the step to eat it.

Throughout June and July I spent an hour or two each day in my garden, puttering when I felt tired, but feeling stronger each week with more exercise and relaxation. I tilled out early lettuce and planted carrots and spinach. I picked green beans and tomatoes and laid them out the length of my kitchen cabinets as if I were setting up an art show. This would be the first summer since my marriage when I didn't can garden produce, but just having a few fresh peppers and cucumbers on the table seemed like a major accomplishment.

Before the fall frosts I potted impatiens from backyard and some of the begonias and set the pots inside near the garage window. I raked leaves and put pine needles around azaleas. I collected grass clippings from the roadside to add to my compost pile, dreaming of a bit more garden along the bank below the driveway next summer.

Chapter 18

MOM

Sunday, March 1

The trip to the zoo was less stressful than we expected. Al in his wheelchair, and Charlie in a rented stroller. Seals were most fascinating to him — I guess because he'd love to swim that way. At first he thought they were baby whales.

Charlie fell asleep soon after we got onto the freeway headed back for Chattanooga. I loosened my belt and took off my wig, putting it in the rear window.

"Turn your head again," Mom said.

I was puzzled.

"I think you're getting some hair!" she exclaimed.

I ran my hand over my scalp. I did feel something different, a downy plush.

"It must be a week's growth," Mom said.

When I look in the mirror to wash my face, I have my glasses off. Not surprising I haven't seen it.

After Ted was ready for bed, Charlie was still going strong. He'd had a nap, after all. I got the scissors, and with him holding the individual long gray hairs out, I cut them off. I could see in the hand mirror that my head was covered with white hair maybe an eighth of an inch long. So I'll be white-haired at 51? So be it! I ran my hand over the velvety surface repeatedly in the pleasure of no longer being totally bald.

Ted and I bought this house because it has a lovely backyard with a basement well on the way to becoming a pleasant walk-in apartment. Since my stepfather Al has been growing less mobile each year, we thought it would be nice if we could finish the apartment so that he and Mom could spend their winters with us in Collegedale in order to escape the long months of ice and snow they have in Montana. Before I discovered the cancer problem, they were packing, getting ready to come for the winter.

One large room that would make a comfortable living room with an alcove suitable for a kitchen was already finished. There was a convenient bathroom. We needed to transform one side of the two-car garage into a bedroom. This meant replacing the door with windows, dropping the ceiling, and dry walling. Then of course, the electrical wiring and painting.

Mom drew plans for a small kitchen. We ordered the cabinets and bought appliances. But with all of us distracted with my treatment, everything went far slower than we wanted. Cold weather found Mom and Al sleeping in the still unfinished bedroom, and it was nearly Christmas before it was carpeted and ready for furniture.

Mom was excited when we told her that we had picked out new bedroom furniture, because since we were married, Ted and I had made do with odds and ends discarded by friends. But when it arrived, I could sense her dismay. We had chosen a style patterned after the Arts-and-Crafts movement of the early 1900s—rather austere and unpretentious, yet beautiful.

When I got home from work the day the furniture arrived, Ted was downstairs, nearly finished with Mom's ceiling. I sat down to watch while he put the last tiles into place. Mom kept looking at her new cherry china cabinet, as if she suddenly saw something wrong with it. We went up to take another look at my new stuff.

"Your bedroom set will be here in a few more days," I said.

"Mine won't match this at all," Mom sighed.

I reminded her that she was furnishing her own apartment, and her taste didn't have to match mine.

Friday, December 6

Mom's bedroom furniture came. Red cherry bed and dressers, two bedside cabinets, with some pretty lamps, a mirror, and blue recliner.

Ever since she arrived here in October, Mom has been torn between her need to do for me and my need to do for myself. When I feel weak, she is eager to fix a meal, clean my house, do the laundry. Dozens of times she's had supper ready when I got home from work. Knowing how tired I am, she often brings the food up and leaves it on our table, even though she'd love to sit down and eat with us. We usually have Sabbath dinners together, and she usually fixes the food.

I imagine it's very hard being my mother. I've never taken kindly to being mothered. But, like me, Mom's a firstborn child, intent on taking charge of whatever job needs to be done. She loves me and wants to take care of me. She wants me to get well, while she's obviously afraid I'm going to die. And I guess it's partially the fear that she might not have me for long which drives her to wear herself out doing all her little kindnesses. I don't know what I'd do if she didn't also have a firm mind-set regarding the sacredness of privacy.

Ted's great about keeping up things around the house, but I know he's grateful for the help Mom has been during these months when I've felt like doing precious little more than go to work and meet my medical appointments.

Monday, March 23

Today is Mom's birthday. I knew I'd have to stay at my office through lunch today, so I made a mini-cake before breakfast. I recorded grades and returned papers. Emily came with Charlie for supper. I was sitting beside Mom on her sofa after they left when she leaned back and looked at me critically.

"Your head needs a better washing," she said. There are black specks in the pores as if you're not getting your scalp clean."

"I lather my head with face soap every night when I bathe," I objected.

She changed the subject, a little embarrassed at my tone of voice.

Monday, March 30

"You're getting a lot of black hair like an undercoat beneath the white," Ted told me tonight when I took off my wig.

So I'm going to be salt and pepper, not white-haired

after all! I can feel the added density as I run my hand over my head.

Mom's getting restless to get home to her own house and yard in Montana now that our yard is greened up and flowers are blooming. And Al perks up whenever she mentions home.

"It's still not spring in Polson," I remind her.

She shrugs. "What's a little snow? Besides, I plan to take my time going back. It will be almost May by the time we get there."

✦

Tuesday, April 21

When I answered the phone at my office this morning, I was surprised to hear Clarene's mom in Minnesota. Mom is there visiting for a day or two.

✦

Friday, April 24

Mom called after I was asleep. Clarene's mother died this morning of congestive heart failure. Mom is terribly distressed, because they have been lifelong friends, but she is so glad she decided to stop by for the visit on her way back to Montana. Friends knew her day-by-day plans so reached her with the sad news in Dakota.

✦

Sabbath, April 25

Called Clarene. Her family had not yet left for Minnesota. Her mother's funeral will not be until Wednesday since the family is so scattered.

I think about how during childhood the two of us played and read together while our mothers worked together on church or school projects. It seems impossible that they have grown old enough to die of heart failure. But if Clarene's Mom is old enough to die, I suddenly realize, mine is too. I imagine her behind the wheel, driving a desolate stretch of western highway, exhausted, her own heart choked by grief.

Chapter 19

WALKING OUT OF IT

Sabbath, March 7

Sunny in the 70s. Ted and I walked the ridge behind the house. I wore a straw hat to keep the sun off my head since it was too warm to exercise that much wearing a wig. Even then I got up a pretty good sweat, which ran in streams across my scalp and down my forehead and the back of my neck. Strange how I had never realized that hair insulated my head from the sun and dispersed perspiration.

As we started down the hillside to our backyard, we heard Doug's noisy car coming up the hill on Lora Lane. We had a great visit all afternoon. So wonderful to have him here! He's brown and strong from planting trees and cutting timber. Mom and I reveled in feeding him. He'd been eating, as he said, mostly soup and beans and spaghetti—nourishing food, but boring after a while. My eyes were so sore that it was painful for me to watch a video with the family, even with dark glasses on. My eyes were weepy; eyelids dry.

During the following days my eyes became so sensitive that I often spent several hours each day in bed with a cold compress covering them. I saw an ophthalmologist, who said it was dry eye syndrome, possibly brought on by the accumulating effects of chemo and radiation. I was relieved that there was no infection and gladly accepted artificial tears as a remedy. And I got dark glasses, something I should have done weeks ago to protect my eyes from ultraviolet. With two book manuscripts in progress, I found resting my eyes a real burden.

Sabbath, April 25

Up at 7:00—feel degenerate rising at such a late hour! Breakfast and then Ted and I walked around back to the neighbor's farm and viewed the world from the top of his hill. I liked the perspective. Napped and read until 5:00. Corrected papers from sundown until bedtime.

Ted's a compulsive walker—has been as long as I've known him. He's always believed that if anything is wrong—physical, mental, or spiritual—he can make it better by walking. During the first few weeks after my surgery he cajoled me into walking with him, if only for a couple of miles a day. He'd slow down to whatever pace I could manage and hold my hand on the uphill stretches. During chemo he had a harder time getting me to walk. I just felt too tired to climb the hill on our street at the end of each walk. So he'd drive me down to the college track whenever I was willing to go, often after dark or early in the morning when few other walkers were there.

Cerebrally I agreed with his philosophy. I knew walking was good for me. And I knew that my most important assignment during the coming year was recovery, more important than correcting papers or meeting class schedules or keeping a spotless house. Whenever we talked about it, I said, "Ya, sure." But putting one foot ahead of the other 2,000 plus times per mile was another thing.

But Ted was creative. At first he watched my *Loon Country* video with me time after time to get me inspired about being outdoors. When it was bitterly cold, he took me to the mall to walk in the evening.

He checked out every suitable walking trail for miles around. When it was dry, he took me on the woodland paths. When it rained, he got out umbrellas and took me to seldom traveled country roads with paved surfaces. We routinely left the house on Sabbath mornings before daylight and walked until time to dress for early church. We walked in cemeteries and along the public greenways along the Tennessee River and Chickamauga Creek. He carried juice and snacks and water in his backpack, and we often had picnic breakfasts complete with rolls and hot drinks while sitting on a foggy bank with the sky just beginning to break open with streamers of sunlight.

We walked the Chickamauga Battlefield trails and nearly stepped on a newborn fawn in a grassy field. One Sabbath afternoon we drove to Chilhowee and Ocoee. After college graduation we spent an entire weekend driving and walking through the Smokies. We picnicked in the rain, enjoyed the snow on the crest at Clingman's Dome, and dropped back into springtime in Cade's Cove, taking Parson's Branch Road out south to the highway, fording the creek 18 times.

Thursday, June 4

Rained all night. Read two chapters in book about business concerns for writers.

I had been housebound for two days because of rain, dashing out to walk the loop through the neighborhood once in the morning and once in the afternoon between showers. About 10:00 this morning I decided that even with another shower threatening, I was going up the ridge behind the house. No chance of meeting anyone walking there this early in the morning—and certainly not in this weather, so I wore a comfortable nylon shift and put on old walking shoes. First to the top, the trail only the length of two city blocks, angling slightly against the ridgeside, but mostly up. I rested once, leaning against the white oak two thirds up, then on up, panting hard and sweating, to the top. Walked north along the ridge first to the saddle where the crest trail drops probably 150 feet. Too steep. Too wet, with all the leaves and mud and small rocky rubble. I decided to walk south instead of going down and circling the back side of the ridge and coming up the east side as I usually do.

Rain began as I turned back, first a pattering on the leaves overhead, and then dampening my hair and the back of my neck. I passed the trail leading down to our house and walked faster. By the time I reached the old bauxite mine a quarter of a mile south, it was raining hard. My glasses steamed up. I put them in my pocket. Near things were foggier than just the rain, but as I looked off through the woods, details of tree bark and twigs were sharply focused, better than I'd normally see with my compromising bifocals. To the east the ridge dropped steeply, the tulip poplars and oaks widely spaced with little undergrowth except poison ivy near the path. To the west, nearly all oaks with some dogwoods. I smelled sourwood and noticed shattered lily-of-the-valley flowers floating in the puddles. I scanned the leafy roof above for the sourwood blooms at the tree's crown, but they were up out of sight among the taller trees.

Where the path bridges a three-foot-wide rock rim between the silted-in mine trenches and jumble of boulders miners blasted apart for a vein of mineral, I watched for slick spots, then hit my stride again as the path becomes a road used at least occasionally by four-wheel drive trucks. Now the rain washed stronger than the full force of the bathroom shower on my head, pouring down my body under my shift, streaming down my arms. All of the poison ivy plants at the edges of the road glistened, turgid with water. Seedling muscadine grapes grew thick like overplanted clover in a field. I'll have to remember in the fall to look for grapes here.

Green—green. Wonderful greenness. I stopped at the gate leading to a backyard where the ridge ends above Prospect Church Road. I turned and started back up the easy grade, walking faster to keep from chilling, walking on the grass and soggy brown leaves instead of on the red clay mixed with the finely broken chert.

"I will lift up mine eyes unto the hills, from whence cometh my help. My help cometh from the Lord, which made heaven" and rain (Ps. 121:1). The rain water streamed off my eyelashes and elbows and the hem of my shift. I climbed cautiously between the mine pits, licking my lips, salty enough that I knew, as cool as I felt, I was sweating. Then I was on the level the last fourth of a mile until I reached the path down to our house.

I started down very carefully, settling the left foot before stepping with the right. Water flowed down the worn center of the path. I stayed on the spongy gray-brown mat of leaf mold and rootlets on the side. Nearly down. Only 20 feet from the grassy edge of the yard, I fell too suddenly to anticipate landing. Nothing broken. I just sat down with muddy water pouring around me and pain in my right knee.

I shucked my clothes at the door and went straight to the shower. All day, even with compresses, the knee became more painful.

I tried to write but decided to walk the pain out. When the sun came out mid-afternoon, I drove down to the Village Market, walked a mile, and finally quit gritting my teeth and gave up on that idea. I went home, feeling defeated.

It turned out I had torn a ligament, but I didn't know that for a while.

With summer we visited rose gardens and historic city streets. Anything to keep me walking. And it paid off. I could feel my strength growing. I was doing something to help myself. I was exerting myself, and exertion has life-giving consequences. By the end of July I was walking five to seven miles a day, often carrying three pound weights.

Chapter 20

PANIC

Wednesday, May 20

To public library to examine juvenile storybooks. Read until time to see Dr. McCravey at 2:30. While he was pleased with my progress, he reminded me that taking out the Port-A-Cath now would be unwise since 90 percent of all recurrences of breast cancer come within the first three years, 40 percent within the first 18 months. Further chemotherapy might be necessary. Ouch! I didn't want to think about that. I've felt so good for the past several weeks that I had dismissed the possibility of more trouble with cancer—and additional treatment.

Dr. McCravey explained about the importance of estrogen-blocking tamoxifen citrate, which he will prescribe. Since my tumor was estrogen positive, taking the blocker will inhibit further development of surviving cancer cells or the production of a similar tumor in my other breast. I will need a chest X-ray every six months and will need to see an oncologist every three months. This means I'll see Dr. Davidson in late August and him in December, etc., etc., etc. At least for five years. Just to remind me I'm mortal.

Rhonda had trouble trying to do the routine flush of the Port-A-Cath but finally got the fluid in. Painful and a bit scary.

Picked Ted up at Cravens House and stopped for a few errands on our way home, including an old-fashioned swing blade for cutting grass. It might require more energy to operate, but it won't break down the way the string weed cutter is always doing.

Thursday, May 21
My right shoulder looks bruised with a few little red specks like blood under the skin.

Wednesday, May 27
Walked ridge and wheeled down several loads of leaves to mulch azaleas. A frightening sensation in my heart when it pounds from exertion.

A dear friend died Friday of cancer. Home by college. Mailed cards and gifts for various weddings and graduations. Walked ridge but strange fluttering feeling in heart when resting halfway up the hill. No pain. Mulched part of garden with grass clippings.

Thursday, May 28
From here on out I'm supposed to have chest X-rays every six months to see if any tumors are developing in my ribs or lungs. I took Ted to work this morning and went to Erlanger Hospital. They do this checkup on ground floor in radiology back to back with the Cancer Center radiology, but they don't allow patients to go that way. The more I find out about this hospital, the more it seems to be designed like a maze to keep patients from knowing exactly what's going on. I'm such a straight-to-the-point person

that this seemed nonsense to me.

First, of course, to the information desk in plaza lobby to arrange billing and insurance, then down the elevator to ground. Front X-ray and then side view.

Back to the library where I spent the morning reading two copies of *The Atlantic*, May and June. Especially interested in article on "Gettysburg Address." Ate lunch at Miller Park, two blocks away, instead of walking the mile plus to the waterfront as I had planned, because there was a very cold wind out of the north, and I did not wear a sweater. Back to the library to read copies of several magazines cover to cover to see just what they are currently publishing—style, format, etc.

Picked Ted up at Cravens House. We went to Hamilton Place Mall to walk but decided to get him much needed slacks and sport shirt. Ate at the cafeteria there and then on to Collegedale to evening camp meeting service. The Heralds and H. M. S. Richards, Jr.

When we got home at 10:00, the phone was ringing.

"Hello?"

"Dr. McCravey. I've been trying to reach you all day. A piece of your Port-A-Cath has broken loose and is lodged in the superior vena cava. We'll have to remove it immediately."

I felt a moment of wild panic. "Tonight? Shall I call an ambulance?"

"No, no. Not tonight. Tomorrow. Rhonda will call you as soon as she gets everything set up at the hospital in the morning. And you can come by car."

"What's gotten loose?"

Dr. McCravey sounded more tired than impatient. "Some of the hardware. They'll have to insert a catheter through the large vein in the groin and into the heart."

If he gave me more information, I was too shaken to

catch it. I hung up the phone and tried to explain to Ted.

"I see," he said evenly, the skin around his mouth turning white.

I walked very slowly to my bed. Ted helped me undress. I was afraid to bend over or do anything to run my heart rate up.

"It's a bit scary," I admitted as he tucked the covers up around my shoulders, "even though it's not really a life-threatening situation."

He sat on the edge of the bed, holding my hand as we said our evening prayers.

I'm not afraid of dying, I told myself as I listened to him moving around in the kitchen. But Ted couldn't handle house payments on his salary alone, and he would be in a very serious situation financially trying to pay off my medical bills.

◯

Friday, May 29

At 4:00 I get up. I've had a very uncomfortable night, sleeping on my back and dreaming worried dreams. Dr. McCravey hadn't told me to be careful about anything, but all night I was afraid that any unusual movement might drive that tubing into dangerous regions unknown. In my study I find diagrams of heart in the *Encyclopaedia Britannica.* I locate the vena cava. I get out the owner's manual for my Port-A-Cath and study the drawings there. I am still puzzled about how much of what is stuck just where. I can feel nothing in my heart.

I write goodbye letters to the children and Mom. Rather morbid, I know, especially since this isn't to be a very serious situation. But I'm scared. No, I'm not. Yes, I am. I crawl back into bed and reach my cold arm across Ted's chest.

"We don't have to get up yet," he says, unaware I've been up for more than two hours. We talk until nearly 7:00, and then he goes to make his breakfast. I don't know whether I'm allowed food and drink. Dr. McCravey didn't say. I call the church to ask for the pastors to pray for me, and since Ted is in the bathroom now shaving and can't hear the conversation, I tell them I'd like to have someone prepared to go to the hospital to be with him if anything goes wrong.

Lorabel, our community chaplain, calls. She'll stop by in a few minutes. Rhonda, from Dr. McCravey's office, calls while Lorabel is here. I'm scheduled for 1:30. I may eat and drink. Lorabel prays with us.

"I'll be there with you," she tells Ted as she leaves.

I'm not sure whether Ted is as glad as I am that one of our pastors is a woman.

I call Mom and Emily.

In Erlanger lobby I see the woman I met at chemotherapy during the winter—the one who wore the turban and had Pam hold her hand and talk about roses and spring. She's very thin and looks much taller than then. She has hair now—about two-inches long and very curly.

I sign in and report to outpatient, where they put me to bed. I'm reading aloud to Ted when they come to take me for the surgical procedure. We don't go to a regular operating room this time.

"You'll feel this like a bee sting," the radiologist tells me. "I will numb the area where I plan to insert the catheter."

Almost immediately after the sting, I feel pressure.

"We're in the vein," the doctor informs me. A nurse points to the two screens.

"Watch now."

I see the catheter moving swiftly through my body.

"It's inside your heart now," the nurse says. "See! There's that stray tube from your Port-A-Cath."

On the screen it looks as big as a garden hose. I watch a thin loop emerge from the end of the catheter, circle the tube, and miss it. I'm frightened, but this is interesting. I pray a lot, watching the doctor's efforts almost like a game. Twenty minutes after he began, he has it, and doubled like a garden hose across a wire, it disappears from the screen. In a second the doctor holds it up between his finger and thumb.

"I want that," I tell him.

His hand in its rubber glove passes the piece of tubing to the nurse's hand in its rubber glove. The doctor grins.

"Wash the blood off, and give it to her."

They roll me into my room about 2:30. Lorabel has a prayer of thanks with us. We watch TV for awhile. Dr. Greer comes to say I need to have Port-A-Cath out next Friday since we don't know its present condition. It certainly can't be used for chemotherapy again even if I need further treatment. The radiologist comes by to release me. He tells me I am to remain lying down except for bathroom until tomorrow morning. May walk, climb, do any usual activity tomorrow. Leave at 5:00. Listen to lullabies on WSMC until 8:00. Call Doug and Mom and go to bed.

Friday, June 5

The Port-A-Cath comes out today! The nurse told me on the phone yesterday that I could have breakfast early but nothing to eat or drink—not even chewing gum, she said—after that. No nail polish on either fingers or toes. I wonder why they always say that.

Walked Lonnie Loop twice after breakfast. Left for Erlanger Hospital at 10:00. Surgery in ground floor ambulatory care unit. Nurse asked the usual questions. Each time I come in I have a longer history to recite. She double-checked to see if she had missed anything then handed me two gowns.

"Put on one gown forward and one backward."

Dr. Greer noticed I lifted my right leg with my hands when I climbed up on the operating table.

"I fell walking yesterday," I explained.

He thought the calf was swollen a bit. He mentioned the possibility of another blood clot since this leg has a bad history. He didn't suggest I'm foolish to walk on muddy trails in the rain.

Dr. Greer had me open before I realized he was cutting. I thought he was still injecting local anesthetic until I saw the reflection of oozing red tissue and stainless steel glistening in the incision in the overhead light. He snipped anchoring stitches from the corners and removed the Port-A-Cath.

"May I have it?" I asked.

"If you want it." We talked about James Michener books while he sutured the incision. Four stitches. A gauze dressing with paper tape. No discomfort. To recovery room. Ted came. Out in less than an hour from beginning to end. Carrying Port-A-Cath in a plastic cup with a green screw-on top.

When I got home I aligned the end of the tubing still attached to the Port-A-Cath to the piece removed from my heart last Friday. Both ends were flat with a split up the side, as if the tubing had been pinched and had moved back and forth until it broke, the way a metal wire will break from fatigue. Nobody has any explanations.

Walked the Lonnie Loop once. To bed at 8:00. I was up from 10:00 to 1:00, not from pain in the new incision, but because my knee hurt. Laid out the edge of a puzzle of an Oregon waterfall.

Sabbath, June 6

According to the written instructions the nurse gave me when I left the hospital, I may have a shower this morning and put on adhesive bandage strips in place of the dressing.

We walk to Apison and back on the road because everything is so wet. Ted carries a picnic breakfast in his small blue backpack. We eat in the shelter at the cemetery. Home with barely time to shower and dress before early church. I wear a hat but no wig. I keep stroking my head when I'm at home—so velvety soft like a tiny baby's scalp!

Chapter 21

MISCELLANEOUS PAIN AND SUFFERING

Sabbath, June 6

I'm beginning to leave the house without my wig. I've quit worrying about people who think it's unseemly for a woman of my age and station in life to have such an extreme haircut. The wig feels terrible riding atop the one inch cushion of hair, which is always sweaty, wet as a filled sponge. I'm still not bold enough to go bareheaded to church, however.

Derrick Morris preached on healing. I kept thinking about his sermon as I set the deck table for lunch and brought out the lasagna. I kept hearing his voice repeating Bible promises as I worked on the waterfall puzzle. I tried to nap but kept making new connections between parts of Derrick's sermon, the Bible texts, and my own experiences. My knee hurt badly. I kept thinking about the blood clots and phlebitis I'd had in the same spot twice several years ago. I might have a blood clot again.

I got up feeling grumpy.

"Since you don't feel like walking, let's go for a ride," Ted suggested.

We ended up driving back roads and enjoying the sunset over different hills at the ends of different small valleys until the sky was dark.

Wednesday, June 10

I'm feeling depressed because of pain in knee.

Have been reading for an hour or so—professional stuff about the writing trade. I hurt too many places today. Since Monday when I realized I'd have to stop walking because of the pain in my knee, I've thought too much about how I feel. The throbbing in my knee—which is probably a blood clot; the throbbing in my groin where the doctor inserted the catheter into the vein to remove the tubing from my heart a week ago—which has probably spawned another blood clot; my other knee—which is always stiff and painful. I'm very likely going to be chair-bound with arthritis and Parkinson's disease the way Grandma Godfrey was before she turned 60. My left arm and hand seem puffy—I'll probably require daily treatments with a pressure sleeve to keep my arm from ballooning. Ankles and wrists ache. What's the matter with me?

I have cancer.

Chemotherapy half destroyed me, and radiation finished me off. I'm doubtless dying anyway.

Why worry about crippling arthritis or hereditary Parkinson's disease?

I stop this litany long enough to remind myself that I did get off several manuscripts in the morning mail. And as Ted says when he's not well, "I am able to sit up and take nourishment."

Friday, June 12

Feeling very tearful and distracted again today after a night almost equally divided between sweating panics and chills. Miserable this afternoon while waiting for Ted to check out in a store. Leaned on my shopping cart and wished I were home in bed. I felt this way right after chemo treatments, I thought. Then the light went on. The prescription Dr. McCravey gave me to block estrogen is listed in my book under chemotherapy. When I got home, I called Rhonda.

"Is the medication to blame for all these symptoms?" I asked, rattling off my list:

chills,

aching joints,

swelling in hands and feet,

headaches,

bad taste in my mouth,

tiredness,

depression.

"How about hot flashes?" she asked.

How had I failed to mention that?

Yes! Yes! I described the past several nights.

"Then it's definitely the medication," she assured me. "We hope things will level off after three or four weeks. They usually do. But if you're one of the women who just can't tolerate the stuff, there's a less effective alternative. We can try that. But it sometimes causes similar side effects."

"If things get better, I'm all for any edge I can gain on the cancer," I said. "But if I'm going to feel the way I have this past week, I'd just as soon take my chances on a recurrence."

"Of course," she said. "But can you tough it out at least one more week to see if there's a little improvement?"

Checked *Chemotherapy and You* by the National Cancer Institute under "tamoxifen," where my prescription's brand name Nolvadex was listed.

"Side effects: needing medical attention as soon as possible: blurred vision; confusion; pain or swelling in legs; short-

ness of breath; unusual weakness or sleepiness.

"Side effects that usually do not require medical attention (unless prolonged or severe): hot flashes; nausea or vomiting; weight gain; bone pain; changes in menstrual period; headaches; genital itching; skin rash or dryness; vaginal bleeding or discharge."

Well, some I have and some I haven't—from both lists. So I'll try for another week before making a snap decision. But I know right now that I don't want to trade my usual vitality and enthusiasm, my usual well-being, for a small margin of safety the prescription promises. I've managed chemo and radiation, believing that I was dealing with temporary symptoms. Whatever life I have from here on out, I want it to be the best quality life I can possibly get a grip on, because I have a lot of living I want to pack into every day of it, whether I have a few months, five years, or until Jesus comes.

To bed about 8:00 feeling achy and tired.

Wednesday, June 17

Had severe pain all night. Bad pain in back and legs all day. Took Tylenol analgesic tablets and rested again.

Thursday, June 18

Called Rhonda. Told her I would stop medication, because I thought side effects bad: joint pain, sleepiness, depression. She suggested I try off for two weeks and see if better. Called Pastor Ed Wright to set up anointing.

Monday, June 22

Walked north to rocky tor then south to the creek bottom and back over ridge.

Wednesday, June 24

I pulled three beets from my garden. Peeling them and slicing them after they were cooked, I felt like Job confronted with God's unbelievable concern about the beautiful details of creation. I considered the course of my own anxiety during the past weeks and tried to focus on the deep red concentric circles as I arranged the beets in the serving dish. I imagined the tissues in my knee ligaments under a microscope and wondered if the cells of my body are as beautiful as these patterns in the beet's root. I walked up the ridge behind the house and both directions to the rim. I'm not sure how much improvement there has been, but it seemed my knees are getting more flexible; there's less pain.

Friday, June 26

I was wrong about my knees being better.

Ted had Friday off, so we drove to Greenwood, South Carolina, to Parks' Seed Flower Day. After two hours looking at gardens, we started home through Hiawassee and Ocoee. As the day progressed, the pain grew worse, and I was hardly able to walk when we stopped at an overlook.

Sunday, June 28

I got up early and read Job 1-10. After Ted left for work, I spent most of morning praying. Since early May my determination had crumbled. I felt weak and unwell. I wondered if it would be like this for the rest of my life with one problem leading to another until I'd be overwhelmed.

Monday, June 29

Read Job 11-22. When I saw Dr. Greer two weeks ago, he advised me to see an orthopedist in order to know if my knees were suffering damage from exercises and walking. I also wanted to know if there was a cause other than the medication for all the pain. Talked to Rhonda about tamoxifen citrate.

Saw Dr. Matthews, knee specialist. X-rays. Torn ligaments in right knee. Little arthritis evident. Anti-inflammatory prescription and exercises with hot and cold before and after.

"Keep walking," he said. "The benefits of the exercise far outweigh any harm it might do. You should probably quit walking steep hillsides in the rain." He smiled as he hunkered down and sat with his back against the opposite wall, my folder still in his hand. His face clouded as he spoke.

"This is personal. A member of my family faces what you just experienced with breast cancer. How was the chemotherapy? You were pretty sick, weren't you? Did you spend a day or two in the hospital with each treatment? What about radiation? Were you admitted to the hospital for the weeks you were treated?"

I was surprised he was asking me. But I guessed specialists really specialize these days, and the folder his receptionist gave me stated that he dealt only with knee injuries, mostly repairing sports-injured athletes.

I explained that all my treatments since the first surgery had been outpatient.

"No, I wasn't very sick during chemo. Just a little for about two days after each treatment. And the only problem with radiation was the time it took out of my work day."

"We're going to have to make some difficult adjustments," he said. For a few seconds his professional mask dropped, and he was a husband or son or brother, facing the unknown. Scared.

Back to Parkridge, where I talked to Dr. McCravey. He was ready to leave the office for the day and looked tired and discouraged. I wondered how many grim cases he had handled during the day. He sat down with me in the small waiting room adjoining Rhonda's office and explained my situation as he saw it. These symptoms, he said, were mostly the result of rapidly induced menopause and were not directly related to medication.

"At 51 you're facing menopause regardless," he said. "Since chemotherapy and radiation brought the onset, you might as well get it over with."

"Will the symptoms subside after the normal course of menopause?" I asked.

He made a wry face. "Probably. I don't know. Tamoxifen is so new that we have little information about the long term."

When I'd asked for anointing, I did so thinking that I would just forget about taking the expensive estrogen blocker since I felt it was giving me all these side effects. After talking to Dr. McCravey I wasn't so sure. Then the next day my friend Marietta, who is a doctor in Texas, called. She urged me to continue estrogen blocker. I began to wonder if the blocker was only indirectly the cause for the problems. Maybe the stress of two surgeries and the pain from the fall, added to the extreme hot flashes, had been the chief cause of depression. I decided to go ahead with the tamoxifen.

After prayer and careful thought, I decided I still wanted anointing but that I would pray for the Lord to grant me productive time and mental and physical health to use the time I have, however much I have—a year, two years, five years, 10 years, a normal lifetime. I was not demanding anything, only telling the Lord how I felt and how I wanted to spend my time and the gifts He has given me.

Lorabel and Pastor Wright came for my anointing. I explained my position regarding further treatment, and each of us prayed. Ted and I walked the track later. Felt great.

July 11, Sabbath
Decided to go without a wig today.

The following two weeks I felt more upbeat than I had all summer. I attended a professional conference in Denver and began teaching composition for the fourth summer session at the end of July. Although the program was grueling, I found myself joyous even when I was exhausted.

Chapter 22

FULL CIRCLE

Sabbath, August 1

Visited old Confederate Cemetery near Texaco on Lee Highway. To Chattanooga. Walked Chattanooga's Fortwood area, where the homes wealthy Jewish citizens built about 1900 have been restored. Picnic supper in front of Hunter Museum, overlooking the Tennessee River. A really devastating hot flash. Walked around the aquarium and to Tivoli Theater for the final evangelistic meeting.

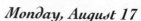

Monday, August 17

Wellness assessment. Walked early. Blood drawn, and all that. One interesting thing was the Body Composition Analysis done with ultrasound on my upper arm. Results showed that if my body were totally free of fat I would weigh 136 pounds and that my body contains 56.7 percent (47.9 liters) water. My recommended maximum body weight is three pounds less than my actual weight—which I am unwilling to record here. I thought all this exercise would bring down my weight, but as the wellness doctor pointed out, muscle is heavier than fat, so while I'm in much better shape than I was a year ago, I am not smaller.

Monday, August 24

Got back report from blood work. Cholesterol and triglycerides are higher than they should be. Otherwise everything is looking good to my layperson's eye.

Wednesday, August 26

Fall classes begin. I teach three sections of College Composition 101 and coordinate the composition program.

Tuesday, September 1

Checkup with Dr. Davidson.

"I see you still have a suntan," she commented as she examined my chest.

She was talking about the two roughly square blocks of skin on my chest that are still considerably darker than the rest of my body. The block from the first radiation set-up overlaps most of the block from the second set-up.

She ran her fingertips back and forth across the long incision scar.

"Looks good. Any bone pain?"

I tapped a spot just above where my breast used to be. "It's tender here sometimes."

"Just sometimes? Nothing to worry about. It's just extra sensitive and easily bruised. Headaches?"

"No. The anti-inflammatory prescription for my knees masks pain. Will it block pain signaling brain cancer?"

Dr. Davidson pursed her lips and shook her head. "If you have a brain tumor developing, you'll feel it no matter what you take."

I pulled out my blood test report from the college wellness program. She nodded and smiled her way down the list.

"Close to the middle of the desirable range. Good."

"My cholesterol is high."

Dr. Davidson grinned as she folded the sheet and handed it back to me. "We have no evidence at present what levels of cholesterol are desirable for women. Tests to establish guidelines have been run on men, you know, and women generally tend to have considerably higher levels than men do. I wouldn't worry about it. You're feeling great and making wonderful progress. Any other questions?"

I brought out my list:

Dry skin behind the left ear. **Should clear up in a few more weeks.**

Ridge in the skin behind that ear. **When dry skin clears, the ridge will go away too.**

Small "kernel" in abdominal fatty tissue. It has been there for years. **If it isn't growing or changing, there is no need to worry.**

Sweats and chills. **These may go away, but then again they may not.**

"I have one patient who's in a dripping sweat every time I see her. She says she's always too warm. She's learning to cope with the problem. Sometimes the body's temperature control system is permanently out of balance after radiation. Sometimes it gets back in balance with time."

"So this may be more than just the usual menopause symptoms?"

"Maybe. Some men have hot flashes after radiation."

Monday, September 21

Ted's Dad arrived on the bus for a two-day visit before he returns to Australia. He's 80 and definitely not aged, although he cheerfully accepts senior citizen discounts on bus fare.

Thursday, September 24

Mammogram 8:30 at Erlanger Plaza Breast Center. Right breast is normal.

Sunday, October 4

Mastectomy a year ago today. Ted and I went on the faculty boat ride on the Tennessee River. Missed it last year because it was the week after I came home from the hospital.

Tuesday, October 6

Saw my surgeon, Dr. Greer. He is more concerned than Dr. Davidson was about my cholesterol. I don't know whether that is because he has more information than she does or because he is a man. I will eliminate cheese from my diet and drink only small amounts of skim milk just to be safe.

Sabbath, October 17

Hunting Island, South Carolina. We came here the first summer we were married and camped with a drop cloth draped like an awning over the back of our Falcon station wagon. That was July — so hot we were sunburned through our clothes. Terrible mosquitoes at night when we slept with the back open.

Early this morning a deer's eyes reflected our headlights as we drove down the road while looking for the beach turnoff. Missed it and had to come back to it. The visitor's center was still locked, and the floodlights gleamed surreally on the pool with a fountain in the middle. A sign informed us that this was the place to observe alligators, but now nothing stirred the green plant film outside the fountain's spray.

This time the weather was cool, almost chilly with the breeze coming off the water, and as long as we stayed out there in the wind, we escaped the mosquitoes still vengeful under the pines and palms. No hardship. We stood on the beach, watching the sky, confused about the directions in the darkness, and thinking we faced west even though we faced the ocean. Then the sky pinked a little above a low drift of clouds, and the world instantly turned 180 degrees for us. We walked along the water's edge, taking off our shoes and letting the waves wash about our ankles, until noon.

Rested. Climbed the lighthouse. Drove some. Returned to motel about 3:00. Napped until 5:00. Read. Ate apple turnovers and ice cream for supper.

Chapter 23

REFLECTIONS ON NOW

When someone dies, we have a funeral. We make time to talk about the person we've lost and publicly to address our loss and come to terms with it. I think that breast cancer terrifies many women because it's such a secret thing.

We go to the hospital. We lose a breast—wake up with that part gone forever—and then we go home to prothesis catalogues or listen to medical fantasies about reconstruction, trying to carry on as if we've lost nothing at all.

I have talked about my loss—a lot. That's been an important part of my recovery. But it's been a moral crusade for me as well. If statistics prove consistent, between five and 10 of my female students from any given year will develop breast cancer. Some of them will die because they don't know anything's wrong or because they fear that losing a breast means losing love. Between five and 10 of the young men in my classes will be married to women who get breast cancer. Some of them will panic. Some of them will run away, afraid they'll be unable to respond sexually to a woman who is "deformed." I've had a chance to show them one day at a time what breast cancer is like—bad, but not terrible.

One of my colleagues on the faculty embarrassed me when he called me a gallant lady, adding a few more carefully selected words, all as flattering, to describe my courage. My students said a lot of nice things to me. And their sweet comments helped me a great deal. But none of them called me gallant. Most of them didn't say a thing about my courage. I don't suppose they thought I had much. Other teachers saw me in my public role. But my students saw me at my weakest. I have never had much confidence in the theory that teachers should "look professional." As if competence were an outfit to put on like a suit and tie to look good in the classroom. Competence is something I am. A teacher is what I am. I am, furthermore, a woman — human.

Every day during treatment I reported in one or two sentences at the beginning of class:

"I feel weak today. Let me sit down."

"You all smell terrible. I love you. But you smell like a bad chemical spill."

"I'm glad this weekend is over. I feel better now."

"My chest is turning pink from radiation."

"They tattooed me today with five permanent reference dots in the case the cancer comes back and I need more treatments."

"I'm blistered."

"I'm burned."

And in August registration: "Look, everybody! Real hair!"

At the beginning of nearly every class period my prayer included my gratitude for these students and their support.

Thursday, December 31

Lying in bed last night waiting for sleep, I thought about where the Lord has led us through the past few years. Teaching college English was never part of my dreams for the future. He dropped the mantle upon me unexpectedly, and I was really quite startled when it fit. Living in town was a thing that both Ted and I vowed we would never consider. Yet after a year and a half in this house, we feel at home. We were never really of the "flee-to-the-mountains-now-and-avoid-the-last-minute-rush-at-the-time-of-trouble" camp. We just cherished our privacy and relished a simple lifestyle.

I have always loved the Bible. As my children entered their teens, I learned as many parents do to pray my way through it with a new intensity—grasping an idea and wrestling with it until I knew what God intended me to learn in this reading.

Once several years ago after struggling with resentment and resistance to change, I prayed, "OK, Lord. So I need more than Band-Aid strips and aspirin. You want me to sign? All right. You can discipline me any way You want to—take away anything I have. I'm giving you permission for major surgery or even amputation. Go ahead and cut."

My pulse quickened momentarily, but after the first flush of fear, I finished the prayer, feeling relieved. I wrote the date in the back of my Bible and waited to see what would happen.

I told some friends about that experience recently and how almost immediately I plunged into one disappointment, one personal tragedy after another.

"I've never been sorry I prayed that prayer," I said. "But if I'd known what I was asking for . . ."

"You can't believe that God caused all those troubles," one friend objected. "Certainly God doesn't . . ."

"'Whom the Lord loveth, He chasteneth,'" I quoted.

"But God's not like that . . ."

I know that Satan's to blame for sin and suffering. But so am I. And I believe that God is an opportunist, taking advantage of every chance we give Him. I'm almost certain He's disciplined me in ways He would never have done if I hadn't said He could. And I'm a better, stronger person because He's brought me through pain. I have learned to trust Him as I could have learned in no other way.

The Word was made flesh and dwelt among us—breathing, speaking. He spoke and it was done. He commanded and it stood fast. Promises, I discovered, are commitments put into words and given life. Just as God's word has power to make things happen, He empowers me so that my commitment added to His authority can turn a resolution into a reality.

Nearly all the days since I learned of my breast cancer have been filled with the normal responsibilities anyone else has to do—shopping and cleaning, working and paying bills—the mundane mechanics of living. Most of the time I have been preoccupied with my daily list of things to do. I have always been aware I had cancer, but most of the time cancer has been on the bottom of my list of things to be concerned about. Sometimes the big thing was correcting the last five essays before comp class.

I have learned during the past 15 months that there are times when it is safe to quit struggling—even safe to quit praying and let someone else pray for me. Sometimes I have thought about how it was on cold winter nights when I was a child. It wasn't my job to get up and feed the wood furnace. Daddy did that. I could lie motionless under the covers, hovering in and out of dreams, hearing his slippers cross the living room linoleum then slap down the basement stairs. I could hear the wood thud into the firebox and the cast iron stove door rattle as he latched it shut.

During cancer treatment, I had to face the fact that I knew very little about my own situation. I had always trusted God. Now I had to learn to trust the people around me — some of them medical experts, some fellow teachers relieving me of some of my work — my students, my children, my husband.

I had trouble admitting I was tired, that I needed human help, because I had always prided myself on my independence, my physical stamina, and my mental perseverance. It was hard to quit in the middle of a task and concede that I didn't have the strength to finish.

I realized more than a year ago that I was not afraid of dying. I have seen during the months since then that I don't' have to be afraid of living either. I can walk around Lonnie Loop this dark December night, walking faster and faster and puffing out clouds of warm breath on the uphill part. I can walk with Ted's Reebok athletic shoes a little out of rhythm with mine — and not try to match my step to his or expect him to match mine. We can laugh more openly, speak more frankly, love more unabashedly than at any other time in our 26 years of marriage.

Without a doubt, this past year has been the sweetest year of my life. After cancer, I am no longer afraid of the dangers lurking in deep shadows. I came around a dark corner. When the lights came on, I saw cancer crouching there. I looked at it squarely, and now I dare to shut my eyes, turn my back on the room, and go to sleep. No reason to assume that I have to stay awake to tell God what He needs to do for my children or my students. He can manage the universe without my help, although He might be able to do more for me and mine if before I go to sleep I tell Him to go ahead and use His own good judgment.

Also by Helen Godfrey Pyke

Doctor, Doctor

For nearly 40 years Dr. John Hamilton has compromised his religious convictions to satisfy his beautiful, controlling wife. Since high school he has loved her—more than their children, more than personal happiness, more than God Himself. Now, faced with an onslaught of family crises, he realizes that he can't face another day without Christ. But what about Maggie? Will finding his way back to God mean losing the woman he loves? Paper, 124 pages. US$7.95, Cdn$10.75.

The Heart Remembers

A daughter, mother, and grandmother find themselves separated by a painful past. Withholding forgiveness from each other as punishment, they realize that their cherished grudges have locked them away from the very people they love and need most. This poignant story demonstrates how God's unconditional love can free us to forgive. Paper, 108 pages. US$7.95, Cdn$10.75.